Handbook of Thoraco-abdominal Nerve Block

Handbook of Thoraco-abdominal Nerve Block

JORDAN KATZ

Professor, Department of Anesthesiology
UCSD
San Diego, CA, USA

HANS RENCK

Professor, Department of Anaesthesiology
Malmö General Hospital
Malmö, Sweden

LENNART HÅKANSSON

Coordinator

POUL BUCKHÖJ

Medical Artist, Layout

KARSTEN HJERTHOLM

Photo

GRUNE & STRATTON, INC
Harcourt Brace Jovanovich, Publishers
Orlando New York San Diego London
San Francisco Tokyo Sydney Toronto

© Mediglobe SA, 1987
BI Perolles 7
CH-1700 Fribourg
Switzerland

Produced by
PACIFIC PRINT PRODUCTION AB
SWEDEN

Printed by
KOON WAH PRINTING Pte Ltd
SINGAPORE

United States Edition Published by
GRUNE & STRATTON, INC.
Orlando, Florida 32887

ISBN (Mediglobe) 2-88239-000-9

ISBN (G&S) 0-8089-1872-9

Foreword

There seems to be a renewal of interest in regional anesthesia all over the world. There are several reasons for this: Investigations have shown that patients who have undergone extensive operations in which controlled respiration is unnecessary, for instance in urology and orthopedics, are in better condition after regional anesthesia than after general anesthesia. Use of regional anesthesia has also increased in obstetrics. Another reason for its wider use are the reports on the environmental toxic effects that repeated exposures to volatile agents has on anesthetic personnel. Futhermore regional anesthesia may be advantageous in primitive conditions, during catastrophies, and in undeveloped countries, where shortage of personnel and anesthetic material may be a problem. Regional anesthesia has also made progress in the relief of pain.

As a sign of the increased interest in the regional anesthesia two societies have been formed during recent years: one in the United States—the American Society of Regional Anesthesia (ASRA)—and the later one in Europe—the European Society of Regional Anaesthesia (ESRA).

This book is written by two well-known anesthesiologists: Jordan Katz, one of the founders of ASRA, and Hans Renck, president of the ESRA meeting, 1986. Their Sisyphean work contains all current possibilities for the use of regional anesthesia in the thoracic and abdominal regions, including spinal, epidural and isolated nerve blocks. I especially appreciate that even simple infiltration anesthesia as a main or supplemantary measure has received its due consideration.

Is there really a need for new textbooks on regional anesthesia, given that anatomy does not change? Are not the classical works by Braun, Schleich, Labat, Dogliotti, Maxson, James, Macintosh, and Killian enough, as well as the modern works by Bonica, Moore, Eriksson, Bromage, Winnie, and others? In fact the steady progress in medicine through research, new ideas, new experiences, new techniques, and new drugs make every new addition to the literature on regional anesthesia very welcome. There is always something extra, positive or negative, in every paper based on experimental or clinical observations.

This book is an extensive survey of the anatomic studies and clinical experiences of the authors and of the up-to-date literature. The text is concise and instructive, with advice on safety and the treatment of complications. The exellent illustrations by the now famous medical artist, Poul Buckhöj, remind one of the classical technically perfect drawings of the nervous system by the Swedish anatomist Gustaf Retzius (1842 – 1919).

For a professor emeritus in anesthesiology, interested in regional anesthesia, this book makes fascinating reading. I congratulate the authors on this illustrated "bible" of regional anesthesia.

Torsten Gordh

Preface

For the successful practise of regional anesthesia a thorough knowledge the anatomy of the nervous system, of the pharmacological agents and regional anesthetic techniques are of paramount importance.

The purpose of this textbook is to present the anatomical background for regional anesthetic techniques within the thoraco-abdominal region together with our personal recommendations and experience for their indications and techniques. In order to keep the volume of text down and to avoid confusion we preferred to restrict ourselves to the indications and techniques that we have found to be the most useful. However, included is a comprehensive and updated bibliography that contains supplementary data and covers additional aspects. In general, the titles of the listed articles provide the reader with information sufficient for the selection of additional reading.

"Thoraco-abdominal nerve block" is a truly international accomplishment consisting of contributions from a Californian and a Swedish anesthesiologist (who once worked together in Florida), a Danish photographer, a Danish-Swedish artist and friends and colleagues at Malmö General Hospital, all coordinated by a Swedish editor. Let us only hope that the multilingual confusion experienced at the erection of the Babylonian tower will not apply in this enterprise. It is our hope that it will provide the foundation for the safe and successful practise of these regional anesthetic procedures that we have found to be so useful in our clinical practise.

Jordan Katz   Hans Renck

Contents

1. Anatomy

Introduction

Comprehensive knowledge of the anatomy of the nervous system and the relation of its components to various landmarks such as bony structures, ligaments and muscles is an absolute prerequisite for the successful practice of regional anesthesia. We want to recommend that physicians who perform regional anesthesia aim at refining their knowledge by continual reference to textbooks and anatomic models as well as to observations made during surgical procedures. It must be recognized that there are many variations from published anatomic descriptions which might be of clinical significance.

In this chapter a brief description of some important sections of the human anatomy as it relates to the practice of thoraco-abdominal nerve blocks is presented.

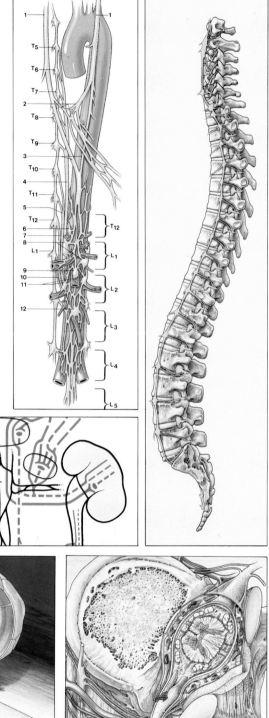

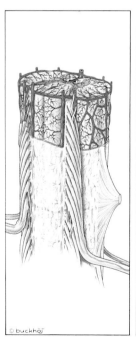

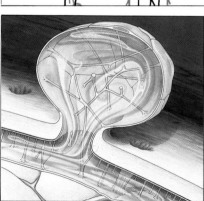

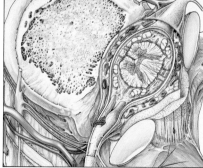

Vertebral column

The bony spinal column consists of 24 individual vertebrae (7 cervical, 12 thoracic, and 5 lumbar), the sacrum, comprising five sacral vertebrae which are fused early in life, and the coccyx, which in reality is the fusion of four coccygeal segments.

A typical vertebra consists of a body (the anterior part) and a vertebral arch (the posterior part). Surrounding the spinal cord is the posterior surface of the body of the vertebra, the pedicles, and laminae. At the junction of the pedicles and the laminae are two transverse processes. The fusion of the laminae dorsally becomes the spinous process. The dorsal spines in the lumbar area tend to be broad and somewhat shorter than the dorsal spines found in the midthoracic region. In addition, there are two small mamillary and four articular processes, a superior and inferior process on each side, attaching to the vertebrae above and below.

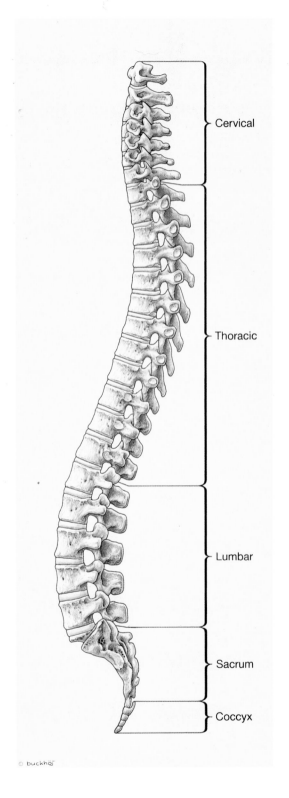

Cervical

Thoracic

Lumbar

Sacrum

Coccyx

Fig. 1.1.   © buckhøj

10

Of interest when performing spinal or epidural nerve blocks are the relative positions of the dorsal spines. The first and second thoracic spinous processes as well as the second, third, fourth, and fifth lumbar spinous processes are in a straight line with their vertebral bodies. From T3 through L1 the spinous processes are angulated to some degree, with maximum angulation occurring in the T4 – T9 area. For example, the T1 dorsal spine is at the same level as its body whereas the spine of T3 overlaps the T4 vertebral body. The tip of the T6 spine is even more angulated, riding over the space between the T7 and T8 vertebral bodies.

Fig. 1.2. Typical thoracic vertebra.

1. Spinous process
2. Lamina
3. Vertebral foramen
4. Transverse process
5. Superior articular process
6. Pedicle
7. Vertebral body

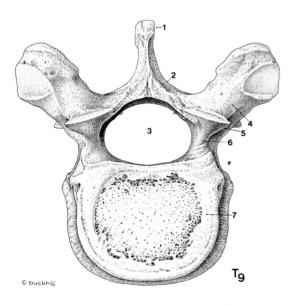

T_9

© buckhöj

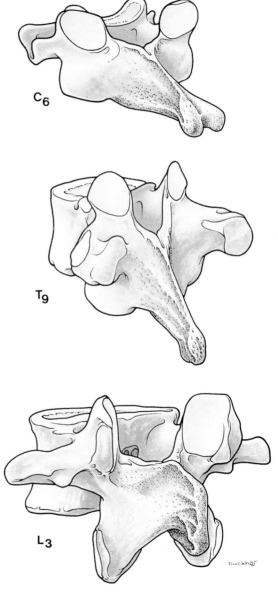

C_6

T_9

L_3

buckhöj

Fig. 1.3. Oblique views of a cervical, a thoracic and a lumbar vertebra.

11

Of greater importance is the relation of the bony anatomy to the underlying neural tissues. This becomes of extreme significance when attempting to perform either segmental epidural analgesia (in the thoracic region in particular) or subarachnoid neurolytic blocks. In the latter situation the object is to destroy the dorsal rootlets of spinal nerves. If one were to put a needle between the dorsal spines of T1 and T2 and into the subarachnoid space the needle would be opposite the dorsal rootlets of T2. However, if one were to put a needle between the spines of T6 and T7 it would be opposite the rootlets of T8 and T9. As a rule of thumb in the midthoracic region, it can be stated that there is a two-dermatome difference between the position of the dorsal spine and the underlying nerve root origin from the spinal cord. It should also be remembered that the nerves which originate from the cauda equina do not leave the spinal canal for some distance. For example, the origin of the lumbar roots is at the level of the T11 and T12 dorsal spines. The sacral and coccygeal nerves leave the cauda equina at the T12 – L1 level.

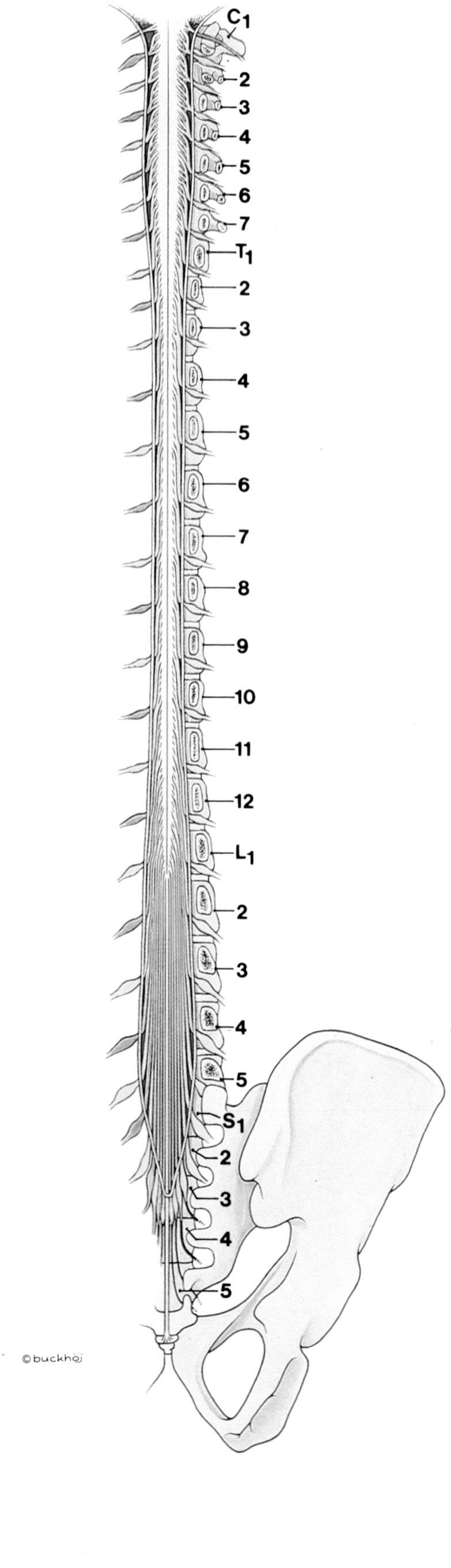

Fig. 1.4. The relation of the spinal column to the nerve root origin from the spinal cord.

© buckhoj

12

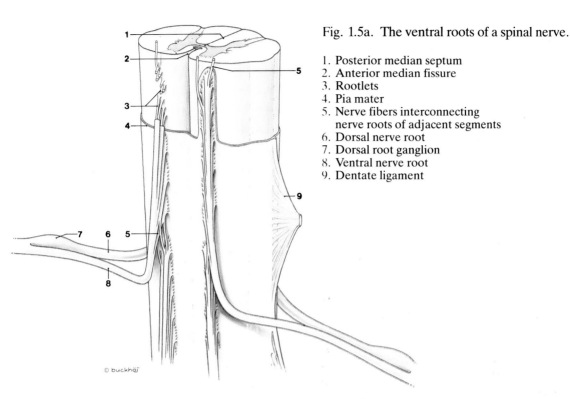

Fig. 1.5a. The ventral roots of a spinal nerve.

1. Posterior median septum
2. Anterior median fissure
3. Rootlets
4. Pia mater
5. Nerve fibers interconnecting
   nerve roots of adjacent segments
6. Dorsal nerve root
7. Dorsal root ganglion
8. Ventral nerve root
9. Dentate ligament

© buckhöj

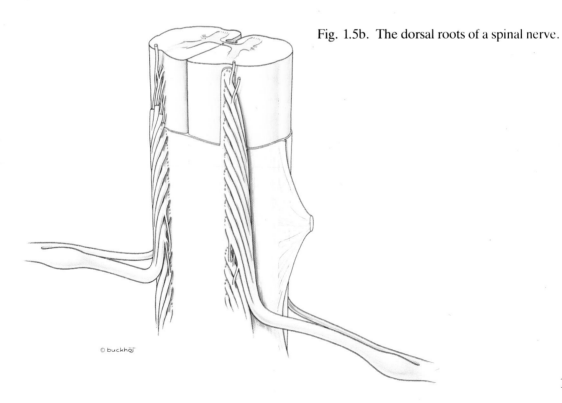

Fig. 1.5b. The dorsal roots of a spinal nerve.

© buckhöj

Sacrum

The sacrum is a rather large triangular bone formed by the fusion of the five sacral vertebrae. It articulates above with the fifth lumbar vertebra and below with the coccyx. From a posterior viewpoint the surface is convex. Down the middle is the median sacral crest which is, in reality, the fusion of the rudimentary dorsal spines of the first three or four sacral vertebrae. It is common for there to be nonfusion of the fifth sacral vertebra, and occasionally of the fourth as well. This opening in the posterior surface is the sacral hiatus. Nonfused portions of the dorsal fifth sacral arch are known as the sacral cornu. On either side

of the sacral ridge exist four posterior sacral foramina through which the dorsal branches of the sacral spinal nerves exit.

From the anterior view of the sacrum, which is concave, one will notice the fusion of the bodies of the sacral vertebrae. In addition there are the rather large anterior foramina through which exit the primary anterior divisions of the sacral nerves.

This is the usual anatomy of the sacrum. However, multiple bony anomalies of the sacrum occur. From the point of view of caudal anesthesia, it is these variations in anatomy that make the procedure less than ideal. The irregularity of bony structures

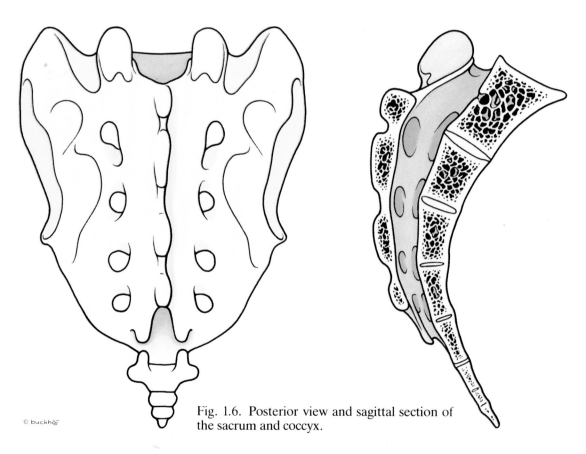

© buckhöj

Fig. 1.6. Posterior view and sagittal section of the sacrum and coccyx.

14

makes identification of the sacral hiatus extremely difficult, if not impossible, and produces a lack of integrity of the sacral canal so that the injection of local anesthetic solutions will not be confined to any particular anatomic space but will rather be diffuse throughout the soft tissue surrounding the sacrum.

These factors combine to produce a significant failure rate in caudal anesthesia, variously estimated from 15% upward.

Ligaments of the spinal canal

The anterior and posterior longitudinal ligaments provide support for the bodies of the vertebrae from C2 to the upper portion of the sacrum. Between the vertebrae themselves are the intervertebral disks, each composed of a peripheral fibrous portion, the anulus fibrosus, and a central section called the nucleus pulposus. The nucleus pulposus is the remains of the embryologic notochord and is most prominent in the lumbar region. The disks are thinnest in the T3 – T7 area and thickest between the lumbar vertebrae. In both the cervical and the lumbar region the disks are thicker anteriorly than posteriorly, which contributes somewhat to the anterior convexities of the spine in these areas.

Of greater significance are the ligaments which exist between the dorsal spines since these need to be identified as one attempts epidural or spinal anesthesia.

The supraspinous ligament is a tough fibrous structure which extends from the seventh cervical vertebra to the sacrum. In the lower parts of the spinal column the ligament becomes both wider and stronger. It actually consists of several layers: a superficial layer with fibers extending over three to four dorsal spines, a middle layer

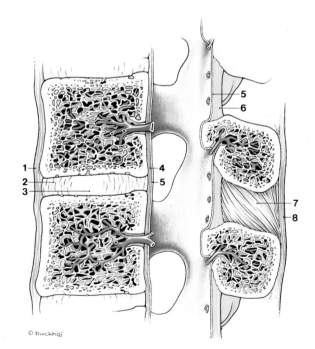

© buckhöj

Fig. 1.7. Ligaments of the spinal column, sagittal section.

1. Anterior longitudinal ligament
2. Anulus fibrosus
3. Nucleus pulposus
4. Posterior longitudinal ligament
5. Dura mater (outer layer)
6. Ligamentum flavum
7. Interspinous ligament
8. Supraspinous ligament

with shorter fibers extending two to three spines, and a deep layer which lies adjacent to the interspinous ligament, between individual dorsal spines.

The interspinous ligament connects the spinous processes of adjacent vertebrae. Its superficial edge is in contact with the supraspinous ligament and the deeper portion comes into contact with the ligamentum flavum.

The ligamentum flavum consists of strong elastic tissue which has a slight yellowish tint to it. The ligament is attached to the anterior inferior surface of the lamina above and the posterior superior surface of the lamina below. It extends from the articular processes laterally to the midline. In addition, and similar to the supraspinous and interspinous ligaments, the ligamentum flavum is both thickest and strongest in the lumbar region.

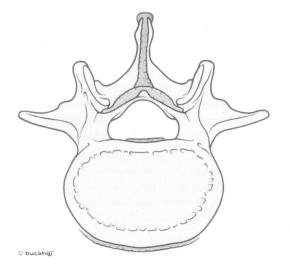

© buckhöj

Fig. 1.8. Ligaments of the spinal column, transverse section.

1. Supraspinous ligament
2. Interspinous ligament
3. Ligamentum flavum
4. Posterior longitudinal ligament
5. Anterior longitudinal ligament

Extradural and intradural spaces

The spinal dura mater is continuous with the inner or meningeal layer of the intracranial dura. It starts at the foramen magnum and continues as a sac surrounding the spinal cord and its neural contents until the middle of the body of the second sacral vertebrae in the average adult patient. This terminal portion is quite variable, with between 40% and 50% of patients having a further caudad extension. At its termination the dura mater invests the phylum terminalae, which is connected to the periosteal surface of the coccyx.

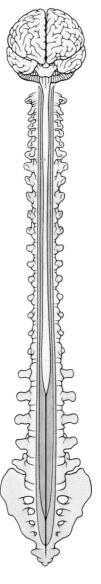

© buckhöj

Fig. 1.9. Schematic diagram showing the levels at which the epidural space, the arachnoid space and the spinal cord terminate.

17

1. Posterior longitudinal ligament
2. Periosteum
3. Nerve root
4. Subarachnoid space
5. Epidural space
6. Pia mater
7. Arachnoid mater
8. Subdural space
9. Subarachnoid septum
10. Dura mater (inner layer)
11. Dura mater (outer layer)
12. Ligamentum flavum
13. Ligamentum denticulatum
14. Dorsal nerve root
15. Ventral nerve root
16. Dorsal root ganglion
17. Spinal nerve

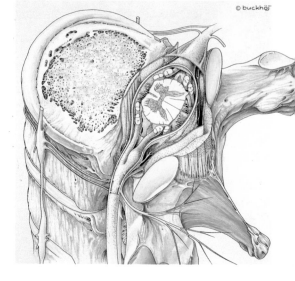

Fig. 1.10. Cross section of the spinal canal at the thoracic level.

Fig. 1.11. Cross section of a thoracic vertebra showing the spinal ligaments and the contents of the dural sac.

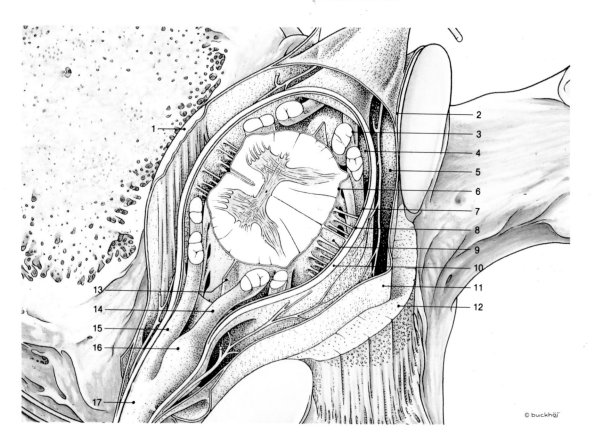

As the spinal nerves pierce the dura each ventral and posterior root carries a sleeve of dura with it laterally. Just distal to the dorsal root ganglion the roots and dura fuse, the roots becoming the somatic nerve and the dura becoming contiguous with the epineurium of the nerve. There are variations in this anatomy however, and it is not that unusual for dural sleeves to proceed laterally several centimeters outside of the vertebral canal. Thus the possibility of an intradural injection exists when performing any nerve blocking procedure near the vertebral canal itself.

Although the dura and the arachnoid act as a single protective sheath for the spinal cord in reality a potential space does exist between them. In fact, a small amount of liquid lubricates the lining between the dura and the arachnoid. It is possible to make subdural extra-arachnoid injections if one is deliberate about the dural puncture and uses a relatively blunt needle.

The epidural space totally surrounds the dural sac and its contents and contains fatty tissue and thin-walled blood vessels.

Anteriorly there are some fibrous connections between the dura and the posterior longitudinal ligament of the vertebrae. Fibrous connections are not found on the lateral and posterior surfaces, although in occasional cases complete septa which follow the fine nerve fibers to the dorsal lamina have been noted. When present these septa might interfere with the distribution of local anesthetics in the epidural space.

Fig. 1.12 Schematic diagram shows levels at which the epidural space, the subarachnoid space and the spinal cord terminate

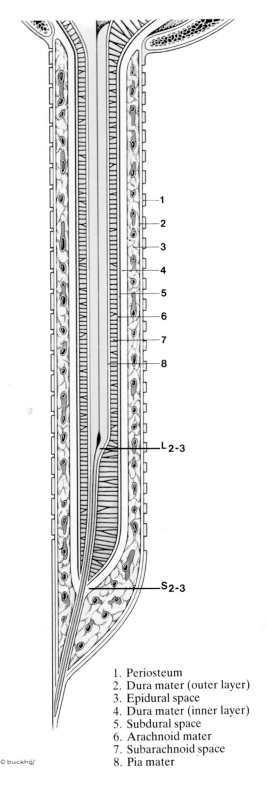

© buckhōj

1. Periosteum
2. Dura mater (outer layer)
3. Epidural space
4. Dura mater (inner layer)
5. Subdural space
6. Arachnoid mater
7. Subarachnoid space
8. Pia mater

19

The actual space between the ligamentum flavum and the dura varies inversely to the content of the spinal canal. In areas where there are high densities of neural tissue, such as the spinal cord protuberances in the upper thoracic-lower cervical region and the bulge in the lower thoracic-upper lumbar end of the cord (in both instances these are the origins of nerves going to the extremities), the epidural space is narrow. Once the spinal cord ends, at L2, the epidural space widens. From L2 downward distances of 5 – 7 mm exist between the ligamentum flavum and the dura itself. In the midthoracic region measurements of 3 – 5 mm of dorsal epidural space have been made, whereas in the lower cervical region the distance may be 2 mm or less. However, if the neck is flexed and the patient is in the sitting position the distance at C7, the normal site for insertion of a cervical epidural catheter, may be 3 – 4 mm.

Fig. 1.13. Anatomy of the epidural and subarachnoid spaces at the thoracic level.

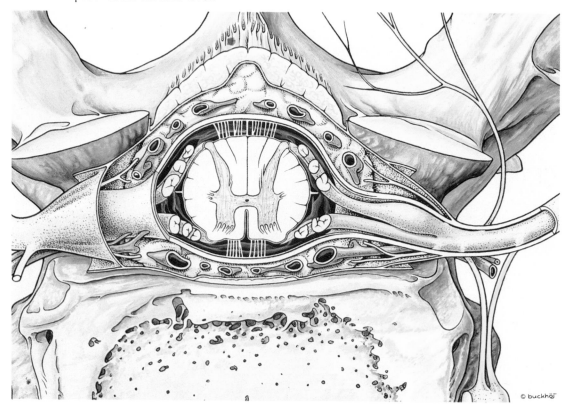

© buckhöj

The epidural fat content is proportionate to that in the rest of the body, with obese people having more fat in their epidural spaces. Although for the most part the fat is free floating, there are connective tissue septa within the more organized fat lobules. In children the fat is relatively less viscous, while in adults it is more dense. This could explain why catheters can be more easily advanced in children. Since anesthetic drugs vary in their lipid solubility, the fat content and the specific local anesthetic agent used will produce different pharmacokinetic profiles.

There are fine trabeculations between the pia and the arachnoid throughout the extent of the cord creating an additional barrier for dispersion of drugs. The dentate ligaments extend laterally on either side of the cord from the pia to the arachnoid, adding some stability to the position of the cord within the subarachnoid space.

Fig. 1.14. Anatomy of the epidural and subarachnoid spaces at the lumbar level.

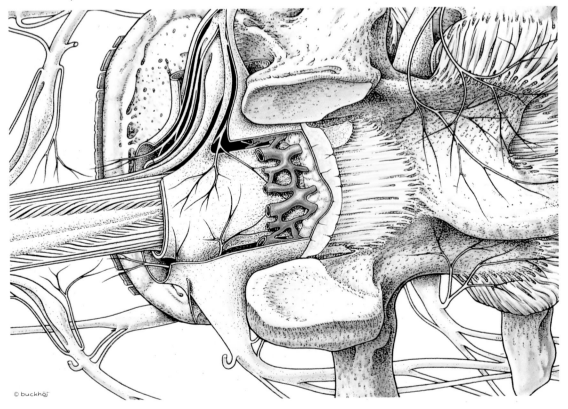

© buckhöj

The subarachnoid space exists between the arachnoid and the pia. Superiorly, the spinal subarachnoid space is connected to the cerebral subarachnoid space. Although approximately 150 ml of CSF is present, the majority of fluid is in the ventricular system, leaving only 25 – 35 ml to bathe the cord and cauda equina. About two-thirds of this spinal CSF surrounds the cervico-thoracic cord with the remaining fluid in the lumbar area.

The CSF is an ultrafiltrate of the plasma with which it is in equilibrium. At body temperature it has a specific gravity ranging from 1.003 to 1.009, the average being 1.005. It exists at close to physiologic pH.

The CSF is formed by the choroid plexuses of the lateral, third and fourth ventricles, the majority in the lateral ventricles. The CSF bathes the spinal cord by leaving the fourth ventricle through the two laterally positioned forminae of Luschka (the lateral apertures) and the medial foramen of Magendie (the median aperture). It is returned to the bloodstream via the arachnoid granulations which project into several of the intracranial venous sinuses. It is believed that this process is for the most part accomplished by osmosis. A small amount of spinal fluid passes out with the spinal and cranial nerves and enters the bloodstream via capillaries and lymphatics in these structures.

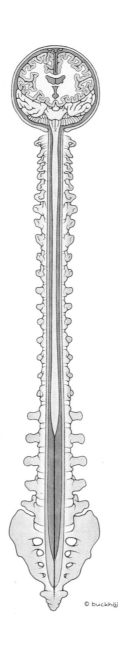

Fig. 1.15.

© buckhöj

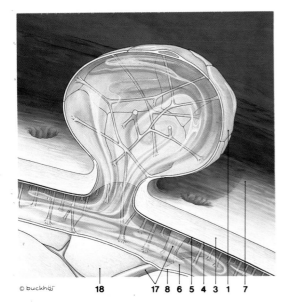

1. Arachnoid granulation
2. Dura mater (outer layer)
3. Dura mater (inner layer)
4. Subdural space
5. Arachnoid mater
6. Subarachnoid space
7. Superior sagittal sinus
8. Pia mater
9. Choroid plexus of 3rd ventricle
10. Great cerebral vein
11. Cisterna cerebellomedullaris
12. Interventricular foramen
13. Interpeduncular cistern
14. Cistern of the great cerebral vein
    (cisterna ambiens)
15. Choroid plexus of 4th ventricle
16. Foramen of Magendie
17. Superficial cerebral vein
18. Cerebral cortex

Fig. 1.16. Anatomy of an arachnoid granulation.

Fig. 1.17. Cerebrospinal fluid circulation. Arrows indicate direction of flow of the cerebrospinal fluid.

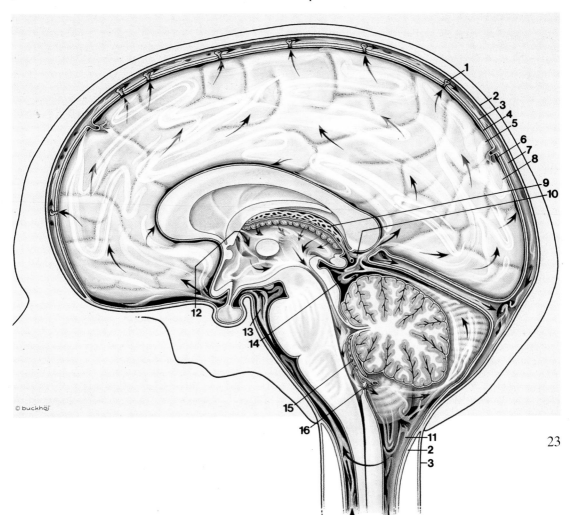

23

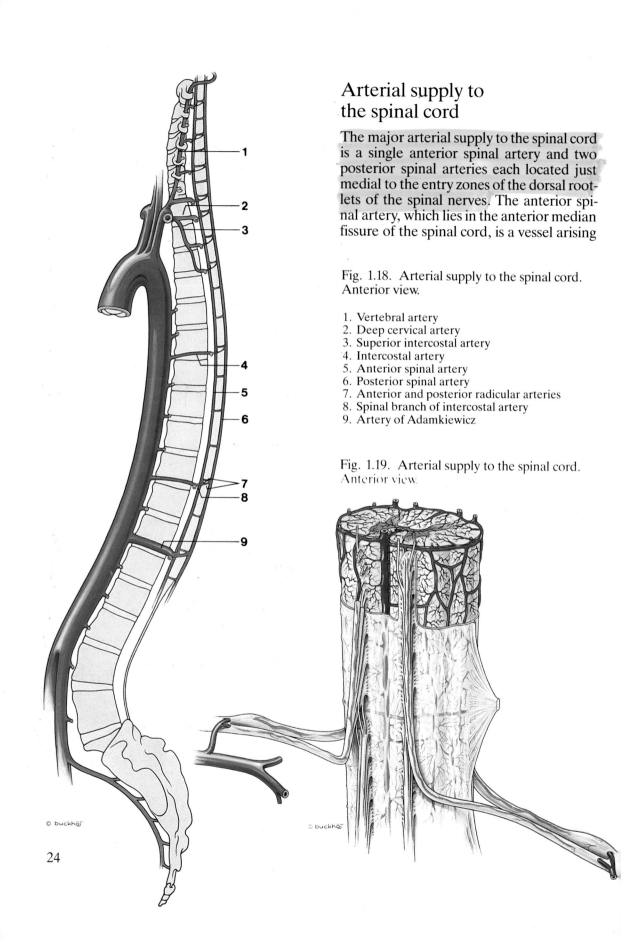

Arterial supply to the spinal cord

The major arterial supply to the spinal cord is a single anterior spinal artery and two posterior spinal arteries each located just medial to the entry zones of the dorsal rootlets of the spinal nerves. The anterior spinal artery, which lies in the anterior median fissure of the spinal cord, is a vessel arising

Fig. 1.18. Arterial supply to the spinal cord. Anterior view.

1. Vertebral artery
2. Deep cervical artery
3. Superior intercostal artery
4. Intercostal artery
5. Anterior spinal artery
6. Posterior spinal artery
7. Anterior and posterior radicular arteries
8. Spinal branch of intercostal artery
9. Artery of Adamkiewicz

Fig. 1.19. Arterial supply to the spinal cord. Anterior view.

© buckhöj

© buckhöj

24

from several contributing sources. In the upper portion of the cord, this artery is formed by fusion of the terminal branches of the vertebral arteries at the level of the medulla and anastomotic channels from the branches of the vertebral, thyrocervical, and costocervical arteries. It supplies the cervical enlargement and parts of the spinal cord to T4. The anterior spinal artery of the midthoracic cord is fed by one or more intercostal arterial branches from the fourth to ninth thoracic levels. From T9 to the termination of the cord there is usually a dominant vessel known as the artery of Adamkiewicz, or more correctly, the major anterior radicular branch. The origin of this artery is quite variable, it usually arises from the aorta between the T9 and L2 level, but occasionally it starts at a higher level.

Variations in the anatomic patterns and continuity of the anterior spinal artery are such that an anastomotic blood supply quite often does not exist from the cervical to the lumbar termination of the spinal cord. This possible lack of continuity means that certain portions of the cord are limited to the blood supply from a single end artery, i.e., the artery of Adamkiewicz. Relative ischemic areas may exist between upperthoracic and midthoracic areas and between midthoracic areas and the lower thoracic cord. Unfortunately, the artery of Adamkiewicz has a peculiar configuration making a right-angled turn within the vertebral canal prior to getting its blood supply to the anterior spinal artery. Blood perfusion through the artery is therefore easily disrupted.

The anterior spinal artery is responsible for the circulation of the anterior two-thirds of the cord via an internal branch which supplies the deep gray and white matter and a radicular branch which sends twigs into the superficial substance of the cord. This radicular branch also anastomoses with the posterior spinal arteries on both sides. The posterior spinal arteries in turn supply nutrition to the dorsal gray and white matter.

Ordinarily, the segmental feeders that supply flow enter the cord bilaterally, however, as stated above, the terminal portions of the cord may be fed only by a single artery off the aorta. This becomes extremely important clinically when certain types of anesthetic nerve blocking technique are performed in the lower thoracic areas where interruptions in the blood supply might lead to ischemia of the cord and to the anterior spinal artery syndrome. This syndrome is characterized by motor paresis in the presence of intact sensation. The onset is usually gradual, over hours to days, but may be sudden in certain cases. Prognosis is almost uniformly poor.

Fig. 1.20. Arterial supply to the spinal cord. Posterior view.

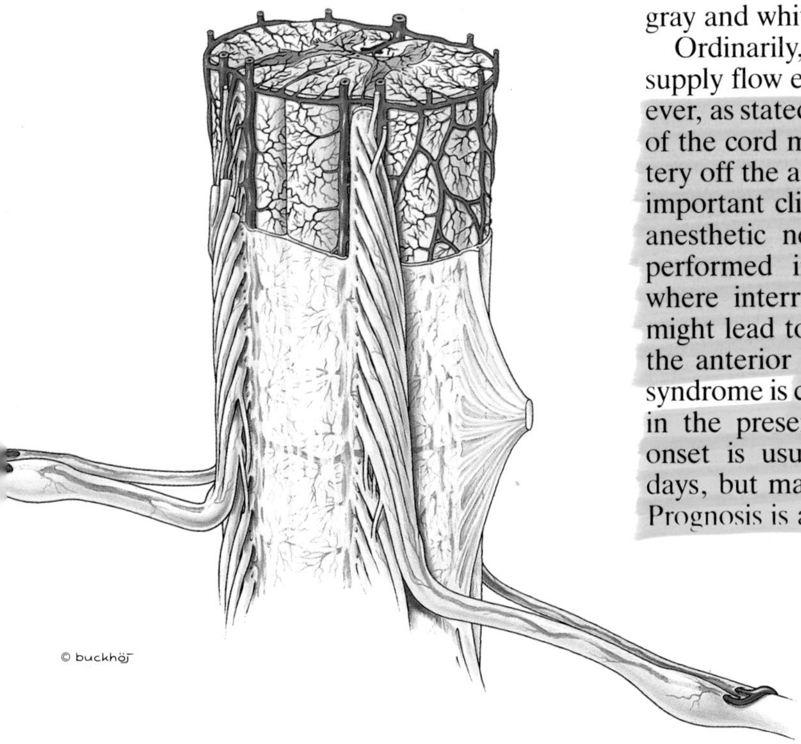

© buckhoj

Venous drainage of the epidural space

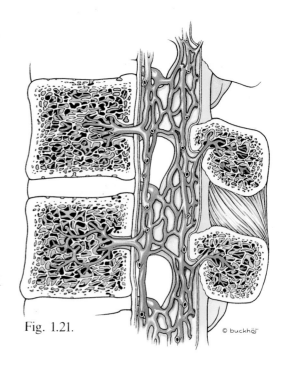

Fig. 1.21.

© buckhöj

The epidural venous system is a complex series of plexuses running the length of the entire spinal canal. Although these circumferentially surround the dural sac and its contents, they are most prominent along the anterior lateral aspects of the epidural space. The epidural venous plexus drains not only the cord and vertebral canal but also a small portion of the CSF via the arachnoid granulations.

At its upper end the epidural plexus communicates directly with venous sinuses at the base of the brain. Below the venous blood drains to the interior vena cava via the sacral and pelvic plexus veins. Between these two locations epidural veins leave the intervertebral foramen and via the vertebral intercostal and lumbar veins empty into the azygos system. The azygos vein, which is located in the right chest, flows into the superior vena cava, just before it enters the pericardial sac.

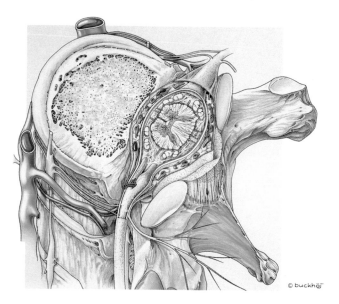

Fig. 1.22. Oblique view of a cross section of the thoracic spine showing the venous drainage of the epidural space.

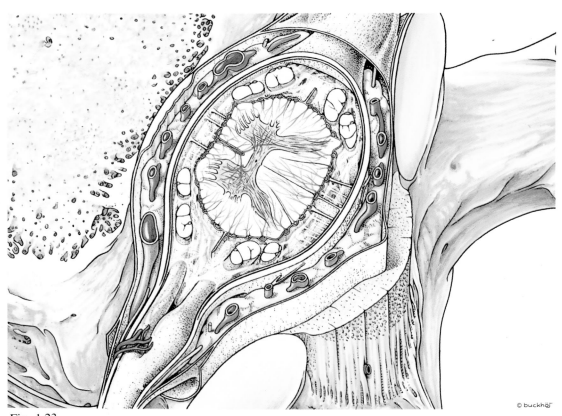

Fig. 1.23.

Spinal nerves

A spinal nerve is formed by the fusion of dorsal or afferent roots and ventral or efferent roots which originate from the cord as a series of fine rootlets. The dorsal rootlets are actually nerve extensions from the dorsal root ganglion, which is located at the intervertebral foramen. Just distal to this the dorsal root is joined by the now fused rootlets of the ventral root to form the peripheral nerve. The dural covering surrounding the nerves becomes continuous with the epineurium of the nerve.

After the anterior and posterior roots of the nerve fuse, and just before it divides into its posterior and anterior primary divisions, a small recurrent branch, called the meningeal branch, returns through the foramen to supply a segment of the meninges and corresponding vertebra.

As soon as the nerve leaves the foramen a posterior ramus is given off. This provides sensation to the midline structures of the back. Almost at the same site the rami communicantes leave in a ventral direction to join the sympathetic chain ganglia (see later text). As the nerve courses toward the periphery at about the level of the midaxillary line the lateral branch arises. This in turn divides into posterior and anterior divisions supplying sensation to the skin over the back and anterior body surface respectively. The nerve then continues to the front

Fig. 1.24. The origin and proximal portion of a thoracic spinal nerve (intercostal nerve).

1. Arachnoid mater
2. Subdural space
3. Dura mater (inner layer)
4. Dura mater (outer layer)
5. Ligamentum flavum
6. Pia mater
7. Subarachnoid space
8. Epidural space
9. Dorsal root ganglion
10. Periosteum
11. Posterior longitudinal ligament

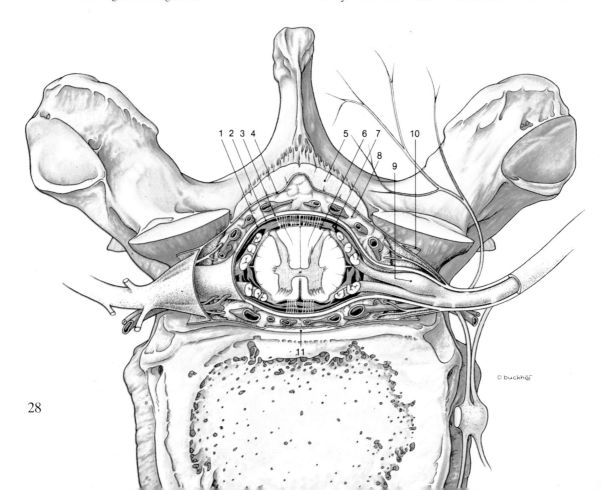

© buckhöj

of the body where its anterior cutaneous branch innervates the midline skin and soft tissue.

The anatomic position of the nerve in relation to the spine and rib is of importance for the performance of paravertebral and intercostal nerve blocks. The main nerve exits via the intervertebral foramen and courses between the pleura and the posterior intercostal membrane. Deep to the rib and about 3 cm distal to the foramen it pierces the posterior intercostal membrane to enter the subcostal groove, in which it stays with the intercostal arterial and venous supply until it reenters the interspace between ribs somewhat medial to the anterior axillary line. The subcostal groove at this point no longer exists and the nerve lies in the substance of the internal inter-

costal muscle, eventually passing beneath the muscle to lie next to the pleura and just anterior to the internal mammary artery at its terminal end. The terminal fibers of the nerve go to the midline and in actuality are thought to supply some cross-innervation about 1 cm over the midline.

Fig. 1.25. Anatomy of the first and second intercostal nerves.

Fig. 1:26

1. Intercostal nerve (ventral ramus)
2. Muscular branch
3. Lateral cutaneous branch
4. Branch to tranversus thoracis muscle
5. Anterior cutaneous branch
6. Endothoracic fascia
7. Posterior intercostal membrane
8. Intercostalis externus muscle
9. Intercostalis internus muscle
10. Intercostalis intimus muscle
11. External intercostal membrane

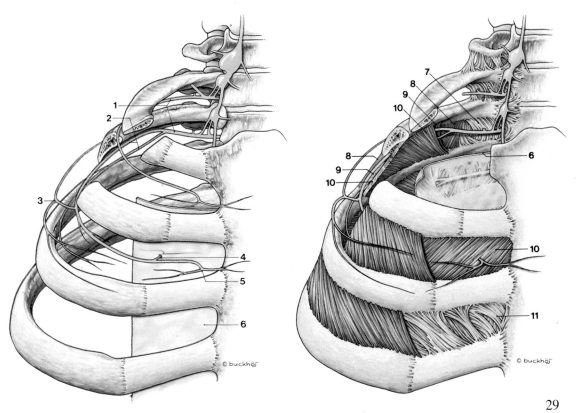

The above course is typical of the second to sixth thoracic nerves. The first thoracic nerve is of somewhat different anatomy. Almost immediately after the posterior primary division of the first thoracic nerve has left to innervate the midline dorsal structures the larger anterior division divides into a bigger superior and a smaller inferior branch. The superior branch enters the groove between the scalene muscles and along with the eighth cervical nerve becomes the lower trunk of the brachial plexus. The inferior branch continues in the intercostal space, where it sends a contribution to the intercostobrachial nerve.

The seventh through eleventh thoracic nerves run courses similar to those described above for nerves T2 – T6 until they reach the anterior margins of the ribs. At this point they pass deep to the costal cartilages and into the space between the transverse abdominal and internal oblique muscles. At the lateral margin of the rectus the nerves pierce the posterior rectus muscle sheath and run within the rectus medially. When approaching the midline they go through the anterior rectus sheath, proceeding to the midline and giving off many cutaneous branches.

Fig. 1.27. Anatomy of the seventh intercostal nerve.

Fig. 1.28.

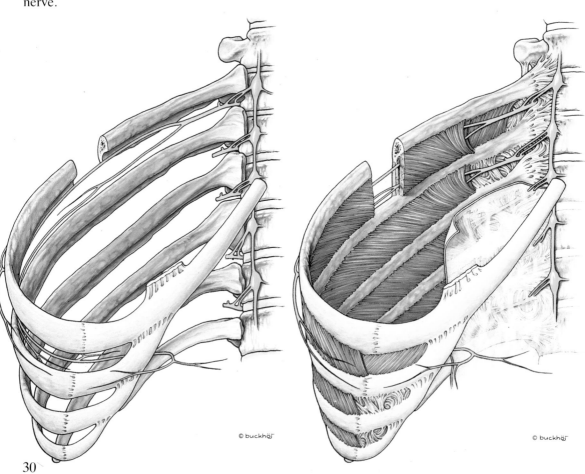

© buckhöj

© buckhöj

30

The skin area innervated by the first 11 intercostal nerves can be summarized as follows:

1. As a part of the lower trunk of the brachial plexus T1 innervates a portion of the medial arm above the elbow.

2. T1, 2, and 3 also supply sensation to a small area of the skin on the posterior and anterior part of the chest wall below the innervation of C4, approximately the middle third of the skin between the clavicle and the nipple anteriorly. In addition these nerves supply the upper inner aspect of the arm and T3 is thought to be the nerve primarily involved in innervation of the axilla.

3. T4 innervates the skin area immediately above the nipple line.

4. T6 innervates the skin over the xyphoid process.

5. T8 innervates the skin over the end of the rib cage anteriorly.

6. T10 innervates the area surrounding the umbilicus.

7. T11 and 12 innervate the area immediately above the inguinal ligament.

The T12 nerve is slightly unique in that it gives off a branch to join the first lumbar nerve before passing laterally. It pierces the transverse abdominal muscle to lie between this and the internal oblique muscle. Branches from the lateral cutaneous portion of the twelfth nerve find their way down toward the skin overlying the hip joint.

Fig. 1.29. Skin area innervated by the intercostal nerves.

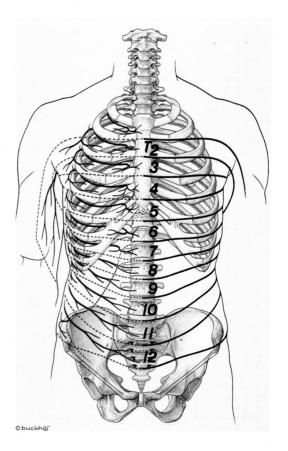

© buckhöj

31

Thoracic sympathetic outflow

The preganglionic fibers of the sympathetic outflow originate in the intermediolateral horn of the gray matter. They pass out with the ventral roots where, at a point just beyond the vertebral foramen, they descend ventrally through the white rami communicantes to the ganglia of the sympathetic trunk. Some of the sympathetic outflow fibers end in the segmental ganglia, anastomosing with postganglionic fibers there. Others pass directly through the ganglia, still as preganglionic fibers, ending in collateral ganglia. For example the splanchnic nerve is a collection of preganglionic fibers which terminate in ganglia in the celiac plexus.

Within the sympathetic ganglia the preganglionic and postganglionic fibers synapse. Some of the postsynaptic nerves return to their respective segmental nerves via the gray rami communicantes, segmentally innervating blood vessels, sweat glands, and the pilomotor muscles of the skin. Other postganglionic fibers may run three to six dermatomes caudad or cephalad through the sympathetic trunks to terminate in more distal ganglia. Still others pass through the vertebral ganglia to end in collateral or prevertebral ganglia such as the hypogastric plexus or cardiac plexus. Some end in terminal ganglia, which are the ganglia found in the myenteric and submucosal plexuses of the gut. It is obvious, then, that the anatomic representation of the sympathetic outflow is quite diffuse and variable.

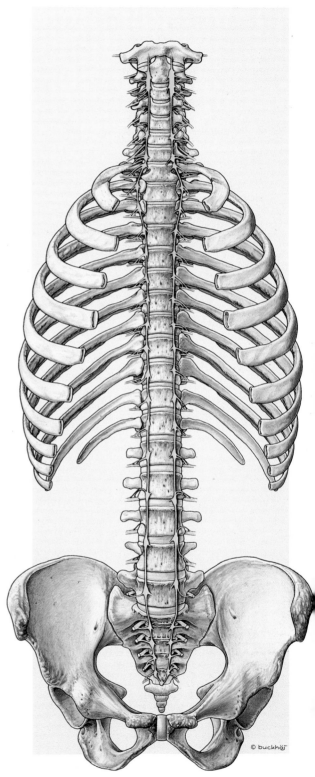

Fig. 1.30. Ganglia of the sympathetic trunk, anterior view.

32

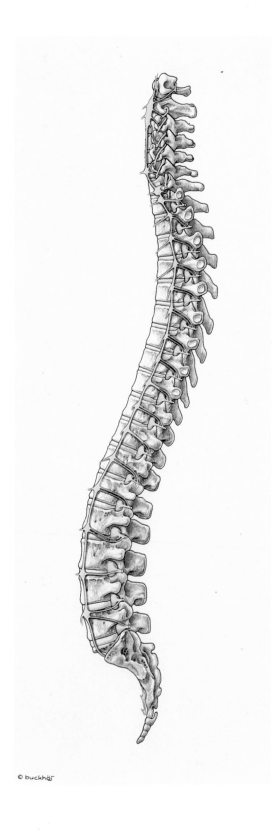

© buckhöj

The position of the ganglia vary depending upon the level of the spinal cord. The first thoracic sympathetic ganglion usually becomes fused with the lower cervical ganglion to form the inferior pole of the stellate ganglion. In general as one descends from T2 to L2 the site of the ganglia moves from just beneath the rib to the anterior lateral surface of the vertebrae. The second thoracic ganglion lies just anterior to the medial portion of the neck of the rib. The next three to four ganglia lie in front of the corresponding head of the rib. The lower thoracic ganglia from T7 to T10 lie just below the rib along the posterior superior surface of the vertebrae. The eleventh and twelfth ganglia are adjacent to the lateral surface of the vertebrae whereas the lumbar ganglia move progressively more to the anterior lateral surface of the body of the vertebrae.

Although the number of thoracic sympathetic ganglia may be as many as 12, usually the first ganglia has fused to become the lower pole of the stellate ganglion and often the twelfth thoracic and first lumbar sympathetic ganglia have also fused.

Fig. 1.31. Ganglia of the sympathetic trunk, lateral view.

Splanchnic nerves

There are usually three splanchnic nerves formed from sympathetic fibers in the thoracic area – the greater, lesser, and least splanchnic nerves.

The greater splanchnic nerve originates for the most part from sympathetic filaments arising from the seventh, eighth and ninth thoracic dermatomes. However, fibers can come from as high as T3 and as low as T10. Individual roots tend to migrate to the anterior lateral surface of the vertebrae where they fuse at approximately the T9 – T10 level. Less than 2 cm after perforating the diaphragm they again become individual fibers which terminate in the celiac ganglia.

The lesser splanchnic nerve is formed from the T11 and occasionally the T12 nerve roots. It lies slightly above the greater splanchnic nerve, between it and the sympathetic chain ganglia. It fuses in the abdominal cavity with the greater splanchnic nerve and ends in the celiac ganglia. The nerve contributes some fibers to the preaortic sympathetic plexus.

The least splanchnic nerve usually arises from T12 and is a small filament which pierces through into the abdomen with the other splanchnic nerves, ending in the preaortic ganglia. Occasionally there is an accessory splanchnic nerve, also originating from T12, which follows the same course as the least splanchnic nerve.

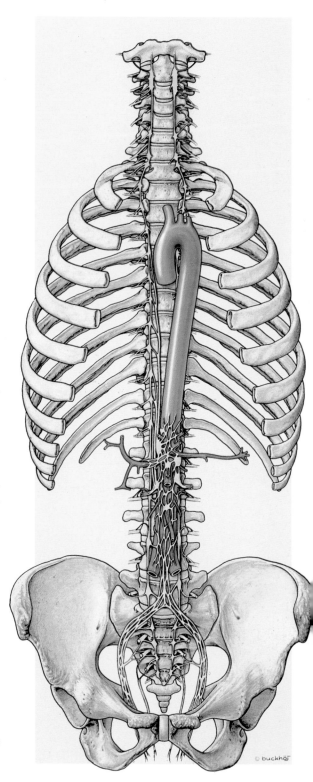

Fig. 1.32a. The origin and branches of the splanchnic nerves.

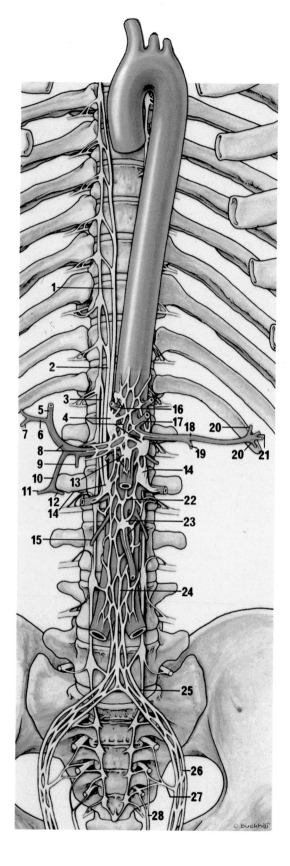

Fig. 1.32b.

1. Greater splanchnic nerve
2. Lesser splanchnic nerve
3. Least splanchnic nerve
4. Celiac ganglion and plexus
5. Left branch of hepatic artery
6. Right branch of hepatic artery
7. Cystic artery
8. Common hepatic artery and hepatic plexus
9. Right gastric artery
10. Gastroduodenal artery
11. Superior pancreaticoduodenal artery
12. Right gastroepiploic artery
13. Superior mesenteric ganglion, artery and plexus
14. Aorticorenal ganglion and renal artery with plexus
15. Ovarian/testicular artery and plexus
16. Phrenic plexus and inferior phrenic artery
17. Left gastric artery and plexus
18. Splenic artery and plexus
19. Pancreatic branch
20. Gastric arteries
21. Splenic branch
22. Abdominal aortic plexus
23. Inferior mesenteric ganglion, artery and plexus
24. Superior hypogastric plexus
25. Inferior hypogastric plexus
26. Pelvic plexus
27. Pelvic splanchnic nerve (nervus erigens)
28. Pudendal nerve

Celiac plexus

The celiac plexus is the fusion of two celiac ganglia plus several smaller ganglia located in the region of the celiac arterial trunk. Although it usually exists as two larger masses lying on either side of the aorta at the origin of the celiac artery, this anatomic description is really a simplification of the many variations of structure which might occur in any individual situation.

The celiac plexus has both afferent and efferent input. The efferent fibers arise from the greater and lesser splanchnic nerves bilaterally, sympathetic postganglionic fibers, the upper lumbar sympathetic ganglia, and terminal branches of both vagus nerves which at the lower portion of the esophagus have become the esophageal plexus.

The afferent fibers are both sympathetic and parasympathetic in origin. Parasympathetic fibers start from the viscera and ascend through the celiac plexus to the esophageal plexuses. Through the vagus nerves they eventually reach the brain and cause such physiologic effects as nausea and vomiting. The sympathetic afferent fibers, also originating in the viscera, pass through the celiac plexus to the chain ganglia or splanchnic nerves on their way toward the cord.

The dimensions of the celiac plexus are quite variable. In general terms it is approximately 3–4 cm in length and 2–5 cm in width, surrounding the celiac artery at the level of the first lumbar vertebra just anterior to the crura of the diaphragm. The right and left celiac ganglia are the two largest components. Each ganglion might be 2–3 mm thick. These are connected by numerous nerve fibers. From the ganglia emanate multiple postganglionic fiber networks to such subsidiary plexuses as the hepatic, prerenal, adrenal, and superior mesenteric.

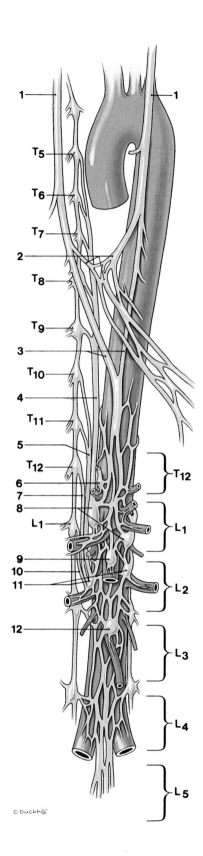

Fig. 1.33. The celiac plexus.

1. Vagus nerve
2. Anterior esophageal branches and anterior esophageal plexus
3. Posterior esophageal branches
4. Greater splanchnic nerve
5. Lesser splanchnic nerve
6. Phrenic ganglion
7. Least splanchnic nerve
8. Celiac ganglion
9. Superior mesenteric ganglion
10. Lumbar splanchnic nerve
11. Aorticorenal ganglion
12. Inferior mesenteric ganglion

37

Vagus nerve

The vagus nerve comprises both motor and sensory fibers. It is attached by about ten rootlets to the medulla oblongata just below the glossopharyngeal nerve in the groove between the olive and the inferior cerebellar peduncle. After leaving the skull, via the jugular foramen, the nerve passes vertically down the neck within the carotid sheath. On the right side the vagus continues its descent posteriorly to the internal jugular vein and then over the subclavian artery as it enters the thorax. It goes through the superior mediastinum, passing behind the right main bronchus to reach the posterior aspect of the root of the right lung. Inferiorly it divides into several branches behind the esophagus where, with branches from the left vagus nerve, the posterior esophageal plexus is formed. From this a trunk is re-formed which remains posterior to the esophagus, entering the abdominal cavity through the esophageal opening of the diaphragm. Once in the abdomen the posterior vagal trunk divides into a smaller gastric and larger celiac branches.

On the left side the vagus enters the thorax between the left common carotid and left subclavian arteries where it passes inferiorly through the superior mediastinum. It travels posterior to the root of the left lung eventually forming the anterior esophageal plexus with contributions from the right vagus. At the caudad end of this plexus a single trunk is formed which enters the abdomen on the anterior surface of the esophagus supplying the stomach and other viscera.

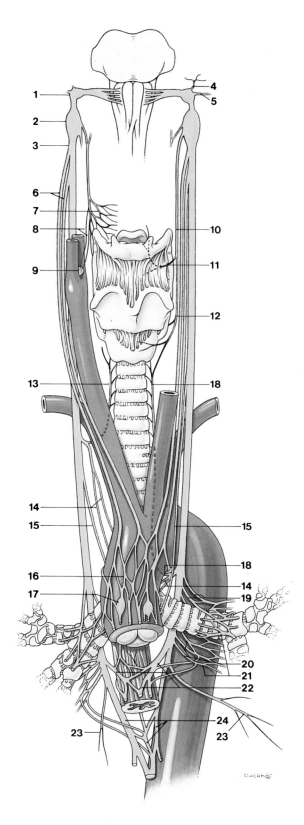

Fig. 1.34. The vagus nerve.

38

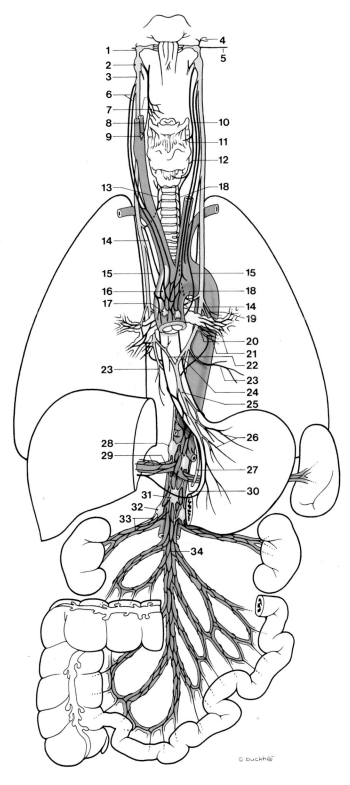

Fig. 1.35.

1. Superior vagal ganglion
2. Inferior vagal ganglion
3. Vagus nerve
4. Meningeal branch
5. Auricular branch
6. Superior cardiac branches
7. Pharyngeal branch and pharyngeal plexus
8. Branches to the carotid body
9. Carotid body
10. Superior laryngeal nerve
11. Internal laryngeal nerve
12. External laryngeal nerve
13. Right recurrent laryngeal nerve
14. Cardiac filaments to the deep part of the cardiac plexus
15. Inferior cardiac branch
16. Superficial (ventral) cardiac plexus
17. Cardiac ganglion
18. Left recurrent laryngeal nerve
19. Anterior pulmonary branches
20. Posterior pulmonary branches
21. Anterior and posterior pulmonary plexus
22. Esophageal branches and anterior esophageal plexus
23. Pericardial branches
24. Esophageal branches and posterior esophageal plexus
25. Anterior vagal trunk
26. Anterior gastric branches
27. Posterior gastric branches (from posterior vagal trunk)
28. Celiac ganglion
29. Hepatic branches and hepatic plexus
30. Splenic branches and plexus
31. Superior mesenteric ganglion
32. Aorticorenal ganglion
33. Renal branches and plexus
34. Inferior mesenteric plexus

Ilioinguinal and iliohypogastric nerves

Both the ilioinguinal and the iliohypogastric nerves originate from the L1 nerve root. There may be a small contribution from T12 as well. The iliohypogastric nerve courses around the body to perforate, at the level of the iliac crest, the posterior part of the transversus abdominis muscle to lie between it and the external oblique. There it divides into the lateral and anterior cutaneous branches. The lateral cutaneous branch pierces both the internal and the external oblique muscles immediately above the iliac crest, providing sensation to the skin of the posterior lateral gluteal region. The anterior branch pierces the internal oblique about 2 cm medial to the anterior superior iliac spine. It then perforates the external oblique and is sensory to the skin of the abdomen above the pubis.

The ilioinguinal nerve, which is usually somewhat smaller than the iliohypogastric, perforates the transversus abdominis muscle at the level of the iliac crest, where it occasionally anastomoses with branches of the iliohypogastric nerve. It then pierces the internal oblique and accompanies the spermatic cord through the superficial inguinal ring and into the inguinal canal. It provides sensation to the superior medial aspect of the thigh, the skin over the root of the penis, and the upper part of the scrotum in the male, and the skin covering the mons pubis and part of the labia in the female.

Fig. 1.36. Anatomy of the ilioinguinal and iliohypogastric nerves.

1. Quadratus lumborum muscle
2. Psoas major muscle
3. Iliohypogastric nerve
4. Ilioinquinal nerve
5. Transversus abdominis muscle
6. Obliquus internus abdominis muscle
7. Obliquus externus abdominis muscle
8. Iliacus muscle
9. Superficial inquinal ring

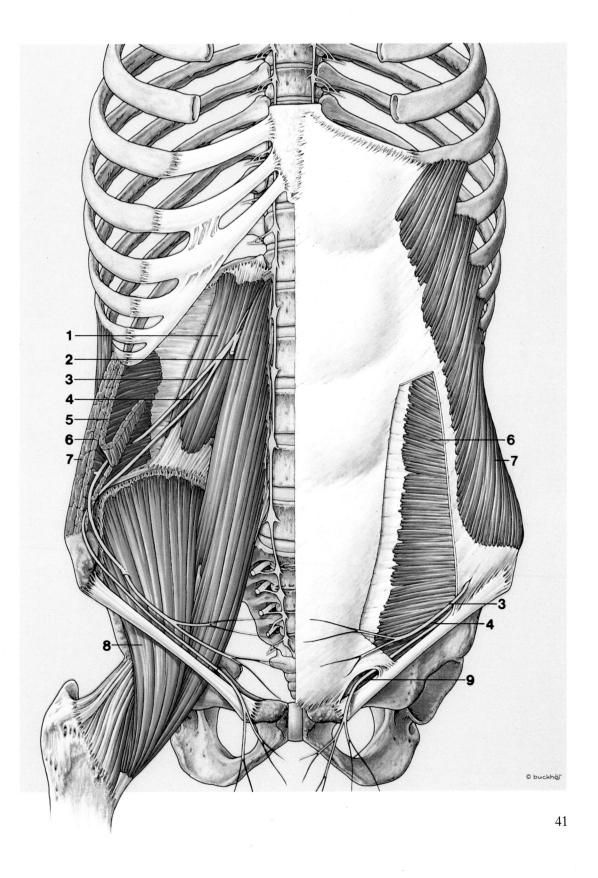

41

Obturator nerve

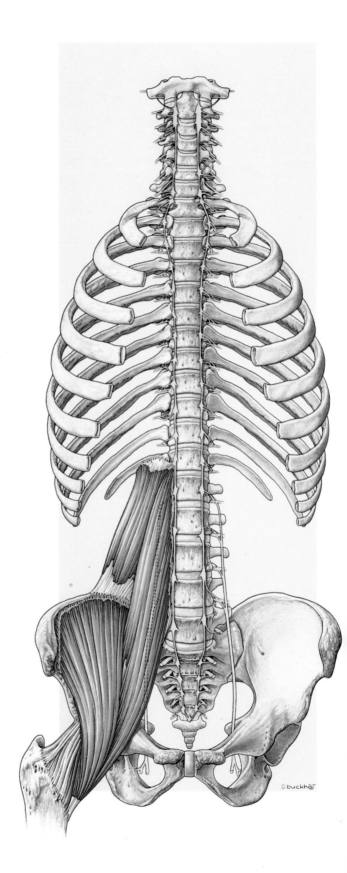

Fig. 1.37. Anatomy of the obturator nerve, proximal portion.

The obturator nerve originates from the ventral branches of L1 – L4. After descending through the psoas major muscle it passes behind the common iliac vessels. It runs inferiorly and anteriorly along the lateral wall of the pelvis. It then passes through the obturator foramen, dividing there into an anterior and a posterior branch. The anterior branch supplies sensation to the skin over the inner thigh and hip joint as well as to several muscle branches. The posterior branch, in addition to its muscular components, sends a small twig to the knee joint.

Fig. 1.38. Anatomy of the obturator nerve, distal portion.

1. Anterior branch
2. Posterior branch
3. Pectineus muscle
4. Adductor brevis muscle
5. Adductor longus muscle
6. Gracilis muscle
7. Cutaneus branch
8. Branch to the hip joint
9. Adductor magnus muscle
10. Branch to the knee joint

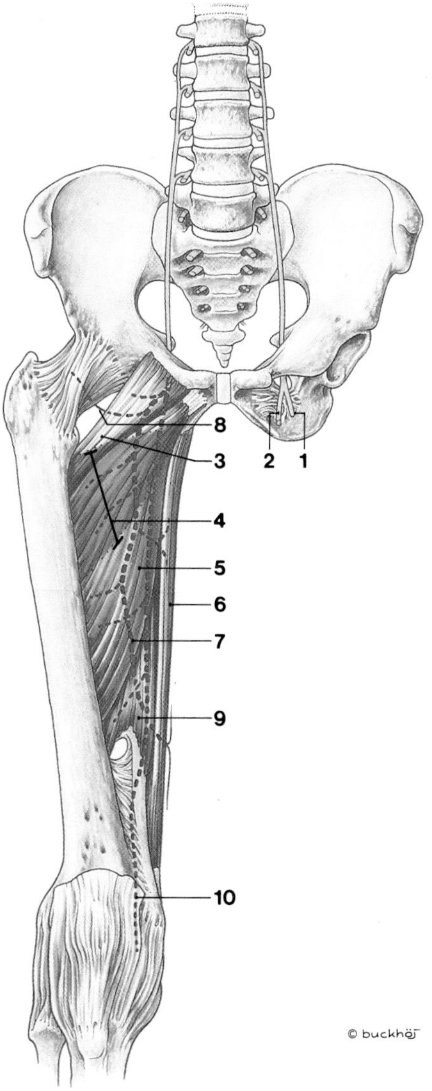

© buckhöj

Genitofemoral nerve

The genitofemoral nerve arises from the first and second lumbar nerves. It descends on the surface of the psoas major muscle behind the ureter, dividing at a variable distance above the inguinal ligament into the genital and femoral branches. The genital branch enters the inguinal canal through the deep inguinal ring and provides some sensory fibers to the skin over the scrotum in the male and the mons pubis and labia majora in the female. The femoral branch ends by entering the femoral sheath, passing behind the inguinal ligament. It supplies the skin over the upper part of the thigh.

Fig. 1.39. Anatomy of the genitofemoral nerve.

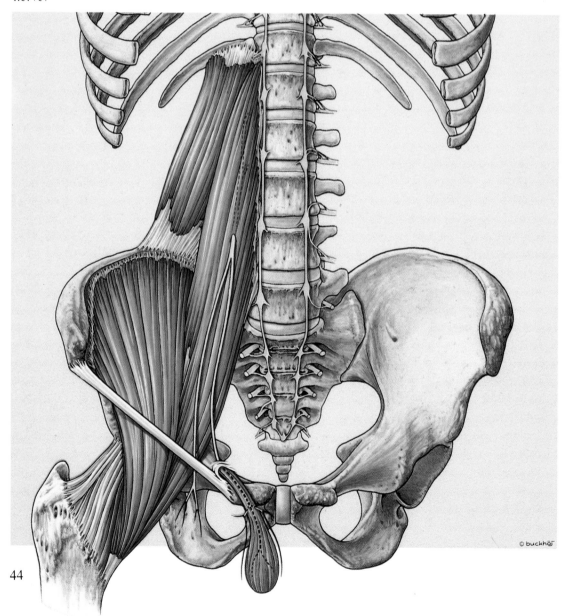

Organ innervation

When one tries to define precisely organ innervation in the chest and abdomen, certain difficulties arise owing to the differences that exist between various texts of anatomy regarding this subject. For example, one text will suggest that sympathetic innervation of the esophagus starts at the T4 level, another perhaps as low as T6. It is often impossible to determine whether sympathetic fibers actually anastomose in the paravertebral ganglia. Moreover, whether nerves to the end-organ are postganglionic or preganglionic cannot be ascertained.

In this chapter we present the consensus of the available literature, which should serve as a fairly accurate description of innervation of specific internal organs.

Fig. 1.40. Schematic diagram of the efferent component of the parasympathetic nervous system.

1. Pharyngeal plexus
2. Superior vagal ganglion
3. Inferior vagal ganglion
4. Celiac ganglion
5. Celiac plexus
6. Mesenteric ganglion
7. Superior hypogastric plexus
8. Inferior hypogastric plexus

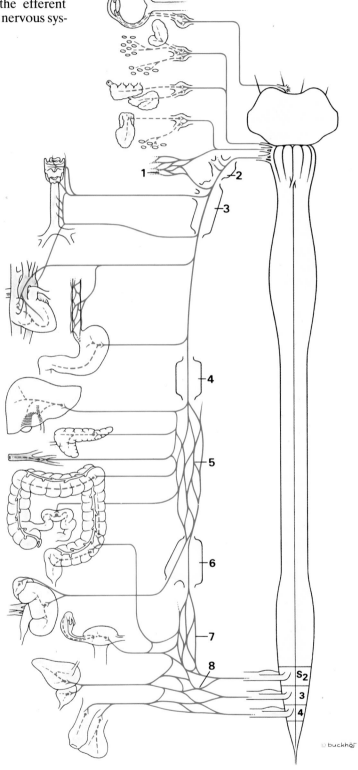

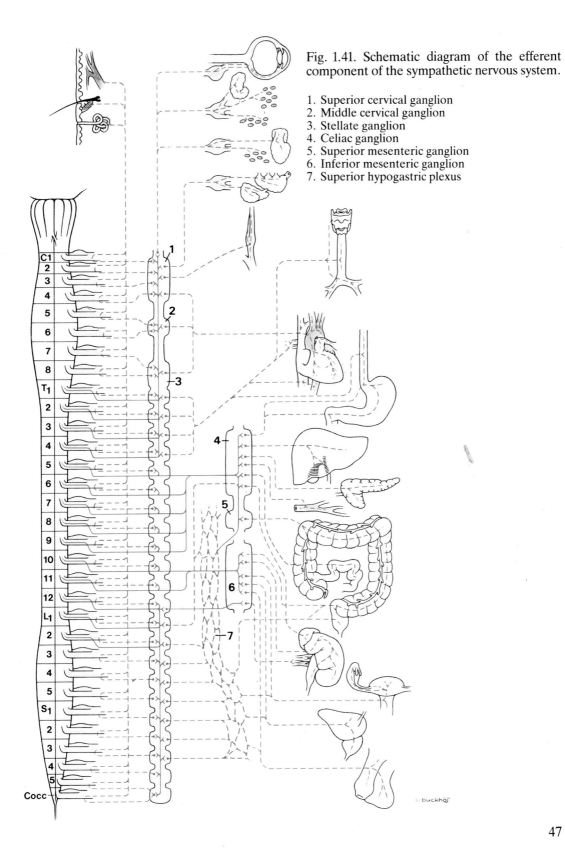

Fig. 1.41. Schematic diagram of the efferent component of the sympathetic nervous system.

1. Superior cervical ganglion
2. Middle cervical ganglion
3. Stellate ganglion
4. Celiac ganglion
5. Superior mesenteric ganglion
6. Inferior mesenteric ganglion
7. Superior hypogastric plexus

Heart

The heart has sympathetic and parasympathetic efferent and afferent innervation. The sympathetic innervation originates from T1 through T4 and possibly from T5. Preganglionic fibers end in the upper four or five thoracic sympathetic ganglia as well as traversing through the sympathetic chain to the inferior, middle and superior cervical ganglia. Postganglionic efferents from the thoracic ganglia give rise to the thoracic cardiac nerves which, via the deep cardiac plexus, enter the musculature of the heart. Postganglionic fibers from the superior, middle, and inferior cervical ganglia form the superior cardiac, middle cardiac, and inferior cardiac nerves respectively. On the right side these nerves also join the deep cardiac plexus. On the left, only the middle and inferior cardiac nerves become part of the deep cardiac plexus, the left superior cardiac nerve entering the superficial cardiac plexus.

The sympathetic afferent innervation follows similar neural pathways with the exception of the superior cardiac nerve, which does not contain any visceral afferent fibers. In other words, afferents return to the spinal cord from T1 through T4, and possibly T5, as well as through the middle and inferior cardiac nerves. It should be noted that visceral afferents do not ascend through the superior cardiac nerve to the superior cervical ganglion.

It appears that the majority of sensory innervation via the cardiac nerves goes to the left lower and middle cervical ganglia, and less to the ganglia on the right side of the neck.

The parasympathetic efferent innervation comes from the right and left vagus nerves. Three branches of the vagus nerve go to the heart: (a) the superior cervical branch, which begins high in the neck, (b) the inferior cervical branch, which is the largest of the three, and arises in the lower cervical area, and (c) a middle branch which comes from the recurrent laryngeal nerve. There are also some small accessory branches from the right vagus where it lies next to the trachea. With the exception of the inferior cervical branch on the left, all of the cardiac branches mix with sympathetic fibers in the deep cardiac plexus. The left inferior cervical vagal branch ends in the superficial (ventral) part of the cardiac plexus. Afferents return over the same pathways.

Fig. 1.42. Innervation of the heart.

Afferent fibers
———— Vagal, parasympathetic
———— Sympathetic

Efferent fibers
———— Vagal, parasympathetic preganglionic
- - - - - Vagal, parasympathetic postganglionic
———— Sympathetic, preganglionic
- - - - - Sympathetic, postganglionic

1. Superior vagal ganglion
2. Inferior vagal ganglion
3. Vagus nerve
4. Superior cervical ganglion
5. Middle cervical ganglion
6. Stellate ganglion
7. Superior cardiac branches
8. Cardiac filaments from right recurrent laryngeal nerve
9. Inferior cardiac branches
10. Cardiac filaments from left recurrent laryngeal nerve
11. Superficial cardiac plexus
12. Deep cardiac plexus

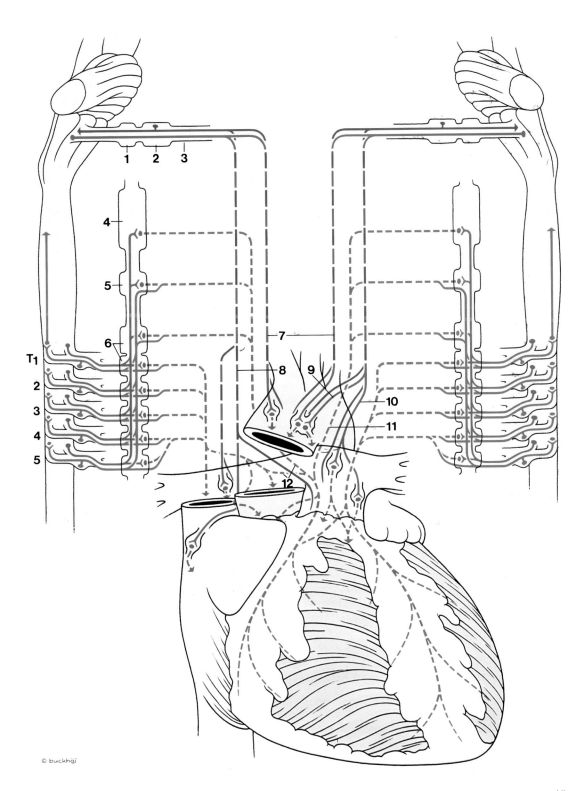

T₁
2
3
4
5

1 2 3
4
5
6
7
8 9
10
11
12

© buckhöj

49

Aorta

The aorta and its vessel offshoots receive innervation from the entire length of the sympathetic chain. Efferent fibers form the various pre- and postaortic plexuses that surround the vessel. Afferents, also through the sympathetic system, return to the cord at specific levels. It has been observed that nerves from the ascending arch of the aorta are derived from the upper sympathetic chain, primarily on the right side, whereas those from the upper thoracic aorta primarily pass to the left sympathetic ganglia. As the aorta decends into the abdomen, eventually dividing into the iliac vessels, afferent sympathetic fibers which exist in the adventitia of the aorta return to the spinal cord via segmental sympathetic chain ganglia.

Pain from the aorta is primarily due to stretching of these sympathetic afferents. However, in cases of aortic aneurysm an additional source of pain might be pressure on any of the somatic nerves.

Fig. 1.43. Innervation of the aorta.

Afferent fibers
———— Vagal, parasympathetic
———— Sympathetic

Efferent fibers
———— Vagal, parasympathetic preganglionic
------ Vagal, parasympathetic postganglionic
———— Sympathetic, preganglionic
------ Sympathetic, postganglionic

1. Superior vagal ganglion
2. Inferior vagal ganglion
3. Vagus nerve
4. Superior cardiac branches
5. Superior cervical ganglion
6. Middle cervical ganglion
7. Stellate ganglion
8. External carotic nerve
9. Internal carotic nerve
10. Cardiac branches of cervical ganglia
11. Greater splanchnic nerve
12. Lesser splanchnic nerve
13. Least splanchnic nerve
14. Celiac ganglion
15. Superior mesenteric ganglion
16. Inferior mesenteric ganglion

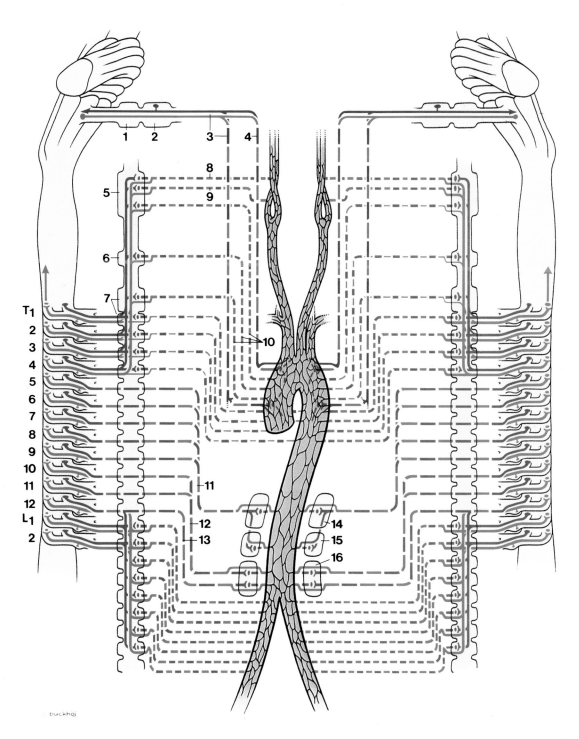

Lung

It must be remembered that each lung receives not only parasympathetic and sympathetic innervation from the same side of the body but also cross-over fibers from the opposite side. Sympathetic preganglionic neurons start in the cord at the T1-T4 level. They enter the thoracic paravertebral or inferior cervical ganglia. Postganglionic branches proceed to the anterior and posterior pulmonary plexuses from which the terminal fibers spread out along the bronchi and vasculature into the parenchyma of the lung. Afferent sympathetic fibers traverse the same pathway back to the spinal cord.

Parasympathetic efferent fibers consist of anterior and posterior bronchial branches of the vagus nerve which arise in the upper mediastinum. The anterior branches are relatively small compared with the posterior ones and pass over the root of the lung into the small anterior pulmonary plexus. The posterior branches, larger and more numerous, join sympathetic fibers to form the bigger posterior pulmonary plexus. It is from these plexuses that the nerves pass with the smaller airways into the substance of the lung.

The lung tissue itself is insensitive to pain, as is the visceral pleura. Exceptions to this generalization occur when fine nerve fibers of the sympathetic system surrounding vessels or airways are pathologically stretched or injured, in which case pain can be referred to any areas receiving innervation from the T1 through T4 dermatomes.

The parietal pleura is innervated by thoracic somatic nerves and part of the pleura overlying the diaphragm has some innervation from the phrenic nerve.

Fig. 1.44. Innervation of the lungs.

Afferent fibers
———— Vagal, parasympathetic
———— Sympathetic

Efferent fibers
———— Sympathetic, preganglionic
------ Sympathetic, postganglionic

1. Vagus nerve
2. Phrenic nerve
3. Inferior cervical ganglion
4. Posterior pulmonary plexus
5. Anterior pulmonary plexus
6. Diaphragm

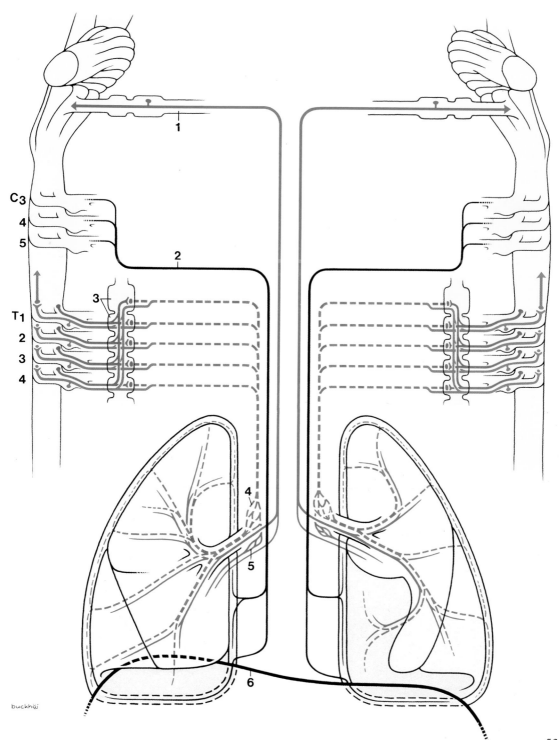

C₃

4

5

2

3

T₁

2

3

4

4

5

6

buckhøj

53

Esophagus

Preganglionic efferent innervation of the esophagus starts at the fifth through seventh thoracic levels. The upper portion of the esophagus receives postganglionic fibers from the stellate ganglion and perhaps T2, 3 and 4 paravertebral ganglia as well. The middle portion of the esophagus is innervated directly by the paravertebral ganglia from the T5 – T7 (and sometimes T8) levels. The terminal portion receives fibers from the arterial plexuses surrounding the left gastric and left inferior phrenic arteries as well as some branches from the greater and perhaps lesser splanchnic nerves.

Afferent innervation enters the cord primarily at the fifth and sixth, and occasionally the seventh thoracic levels.

The parasympathetic innervation of the esophagus is from the vagus nerves. The upper (neck) portion of the esophagus receives branches from the recurrent laryngeal nerve. The left vagus supplies primarily the anterior part of the thoracic esophagus and the right vagus the posterior part, although fibers from both intermingle.

Fig. 1.45. Innervation of the esophagus.

Afferent fibers
———— Vagal, parasympathetic
———— Sympathetic

Efferent fibers
———— Vagal, parasympathetic preganglionic
‒‒‒‒‒‒ Vagal, parasympathetic postganglionic
———— Sympathetic, preganglionic
‒‒‒‒‒‒ Sympathetic, postganglionic

1. Stellate ganglion
2. Vagus nerve
3. Recurrent laryngeal nerve
4. Celiac ganglion
5. Plexus surrounding left inferior phrenic artery
6. Celiac plexus
7. Greater splanchnic nerve

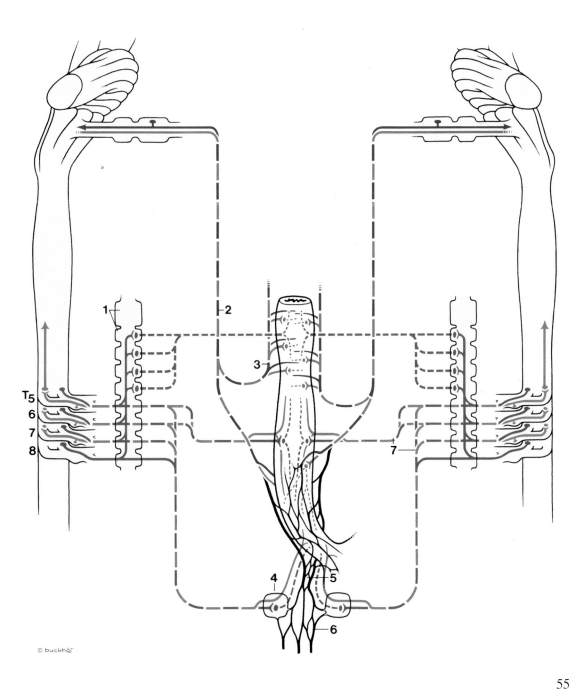

T₅
6
7
8

© buckhöj

Diaphragm

The diaphragm is primarily innervated by the phrenic nerves which are derived from fibers of C4, with smaller contributions from C3 and C5. The phrenic nerves pierce the diaphragm bilaterally sending out an extensive network of fibers on its inferior surface. In addition, some of the peripheral muscular fibers of the diaphragm are supplied by the lower sixth thoracic somatic nerves with both efferent and afferent components.

Fig. 1.46. Innervation of the diaphragm.

Afferent fibers
———— Sympathetic

Efferent fibers
———— Sympathetic, preganglionic
╌╌╌╌╌ Sympathetic, postganglionic

1. Phrenic nerve
2. Intercostal nerves

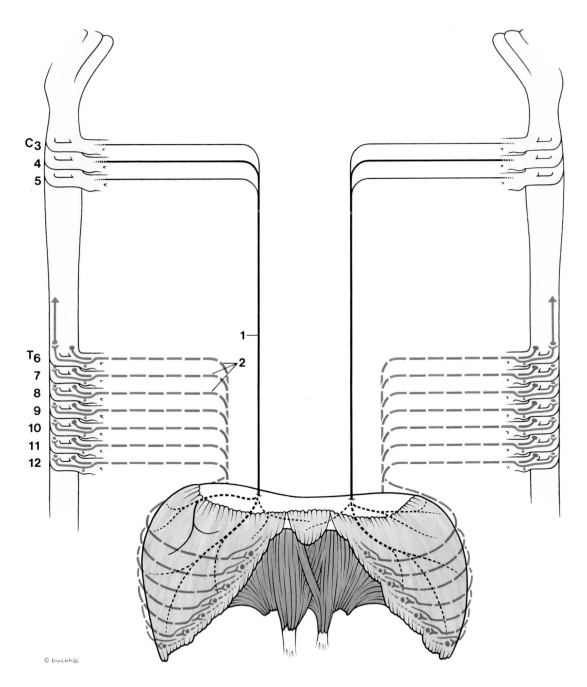

Liver and biliary system

Sympathetic fibers leave the cord from T6 to T9 and travel via the greater splanchnic nerves to the celiac plexus. They then pass laterally toward the liver, forming the anterior and posterior hepatic plexuses. Parasympathetic fibers in the left vagus nerves go directly into the anterior hepatic plexus whereas those from the right pass through the celiac plexus first before entering the posterior hepatic plexus. From the anterior hepatic plexus fibers surround the hepatic artery, with branches terminating in the gallbladder, cystic duct, and pancreatic duct. Posterior hepatic plexus fibers are primarily associated with the portal vein and bile duct.

Since the plexuses do communicate with each other it is obvious that all structures of the hepatobiliary system receive innervation from both, although the major innervation is as listed above.

Afferent innervation of this area returns to the spinal cord through the splanchnic nerves, primarily to T8 and T9, and to a lesser extent to T6 and T7.

Fig. 1.47. Innervation of the liver and biliary system.

Afferent fibers
——— Vagal, parasympathetic
——— Sympathetic

Efferent fibers
——— Vagal, parasympathetic preganglionic
------ Vagal, parasympathetic postganglionic
——— Sympathetic, preganglionic
------ Sympathetic, postganglionic

1. Vagus nerve
2. Greater splanchnic nerve
3. Lesser splanchnic nerve
4. Cystic duct
5. Portal vein
6. Bile duct
7. Pancreatic duct
8. Posterior hepatic plexus
9. Anterior hepatic plexus
10. Anterior esophageal branches of vagus nerve
11. Posterior esophageal branches of vagus nerve
12. Celiac ganglion
13. Celiac plexus
14. Hepatic branch from anterior esophageal plexus
15. Aorticorenal ganglion

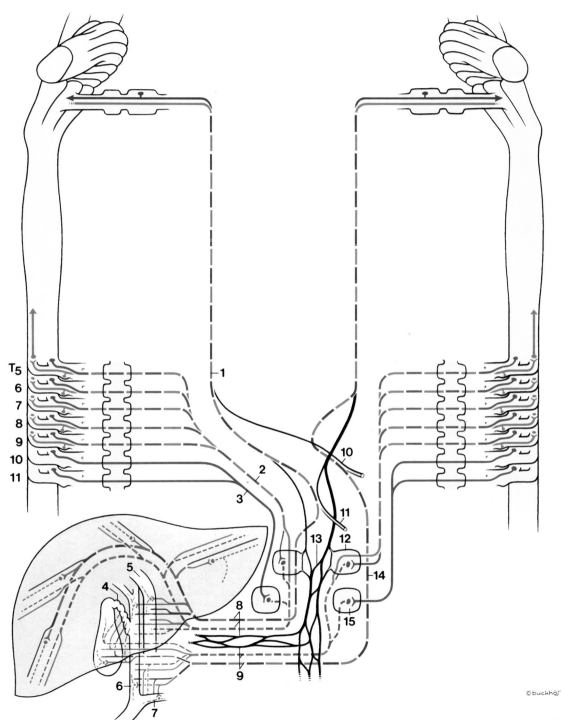

T5
6
7
8
9
10
11

1

2

3

10

11

13

12

14

15

5

4

8

9

6

7

©buckhöj

59

Stomach

Efferent sympathetic innervation starts at the T5 – T11 level and travels via the splanchnic nerves to the celiac plexus. Postganglionic nerves then follow the arterial supply of the stomach to terminate in the organ.

The parasympathetic innervation is from both vagus nerves. The left vagus goes to the anterior part of the stomach and the right vagus to the posterior aspect. The nerves to the pyloric canal and first part of the duodenum are supplied by the hepatic branches of the left vagus.

Sympathetic fibers pass back to the cord and enter it at T7, 8, and 9. Afferents also return via vagal parasympathetic fibers.

Fig. 1.48. Innervation of the stomach.

Afferent fibers
_____ Vagal, parasympathetic
_____ Sympathetic

Efferent fibers
_____ Vagal, parasympathetic preganglionic
- - - - - - Vagal, parasympathetic postganglionic
_____ Sympathetic, preganglionic
- - - - - - Sympathetic, postganglionic

1. Vagus nerve
2. Anterior esophageal branches from esophageal plexus
3. Posterior esophageal branches from esophageal plexus
4. Plexus surrounding inferior phrenic arteries
5. Greater splanchnic nerve
6. Celiac ganglion
7. Lesser splanchnic nerve
8. Aorticorenal ganglion
9. Celiac plexus
10. Hepatic branch from anterior esophageal plexus

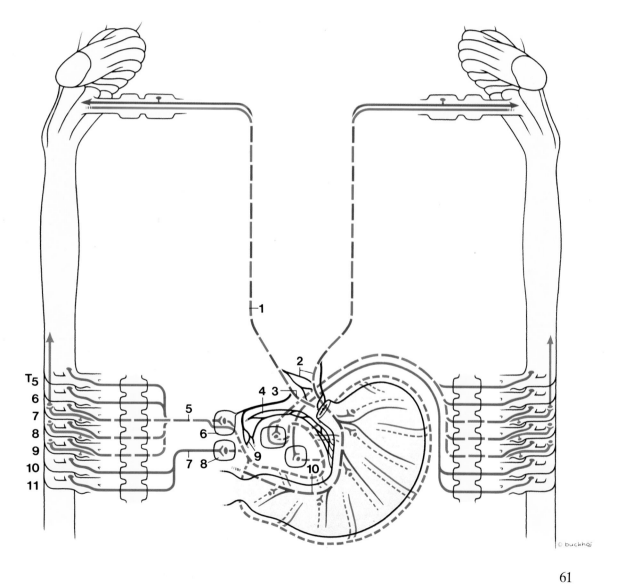

T5
6
7
8
9
10
11

1

2

4 3

5

6

7 8

9

10

© buckhøj

Pancreas

The pancreas has both sympathetic and parasympathetic innervation. Efferent sympathetic fibers originate at T5–T11 dermatomes. Fibers may course through the paravertebral ganglia directly to the celiac plexus or their route may be via the splanchnic nerves. Postganglionic fibers from the celiac plexus pass with the vasculature into the substance of the pancreas.

Parasympathetic efferent innervation is from the right and left vagus, most of the fibers coming from the right nerve. They traverse the celiac plexus and follow the sympathetic supply to the interior of the gland.

Afferent sympathetic innervation enters the spinal cord from T6–T10 bilaterally. In addition, there are afferent vagal fibers.

Fig. 1.49. Innervation of the pancreas.

Afferent fibers
_____ Vagal, parasympathetic
_____ Sympathetic

Efferent fibers
_____ Vagal, parasympathetic preganglionic
------- Vagal, parasympathetic postganglionic
_____ Sympathetic, preganglionic
------- Sympathetic, postganglionic

1. Vagus nerve
2. Greater splanchnic nerve
3. Celiac ganglion
4. Lesser splanchnic nerve
5. Aorticorenal ganglion
6. Hepatic plexus
7. Plexus surrounding gastroduodenal artery
8. Celiac plexus
9. Plexus surrounding pancreatic artery
10. Splenic plexus

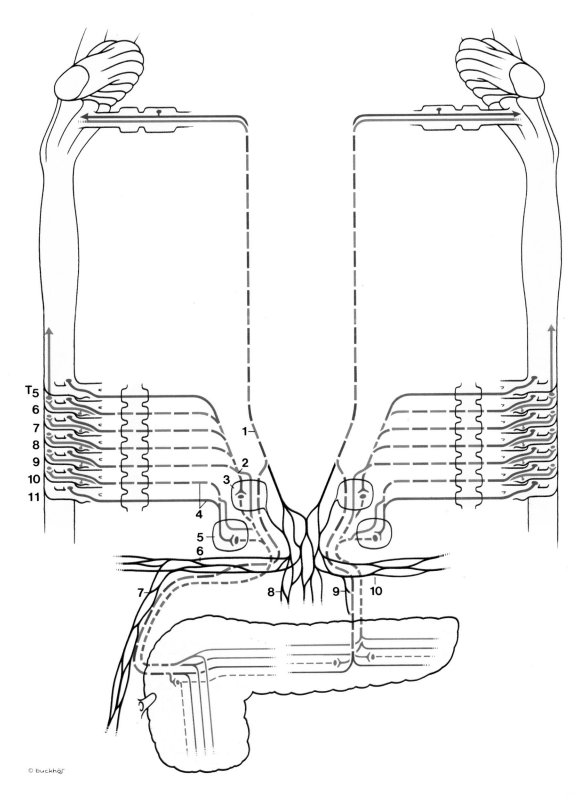

T₅

© buckhöj

63

T_5

© buckhöj

Spleen

The innervation of the spleen is similar to that of the pancreas except that its origin from the cord is more restricted to T6 – T8.

Fig. 1.50. Innervation of the spleen.

Afferent fibers
——————— Vagal, parasympathetic
——————— Sympathetic

Efferent fibers
——————— Vagal, parasympathetic preganglionic
.------- Vagal, parasympathetic postganglionic
——————— Sympathetic, preganglionic
.------- Sympathetic, postganglionic

1. Greater splanchnic nerve
2. Vagus nerve
3. Celiac ganglion
4. Celiac plexus
5. Splenic plexus

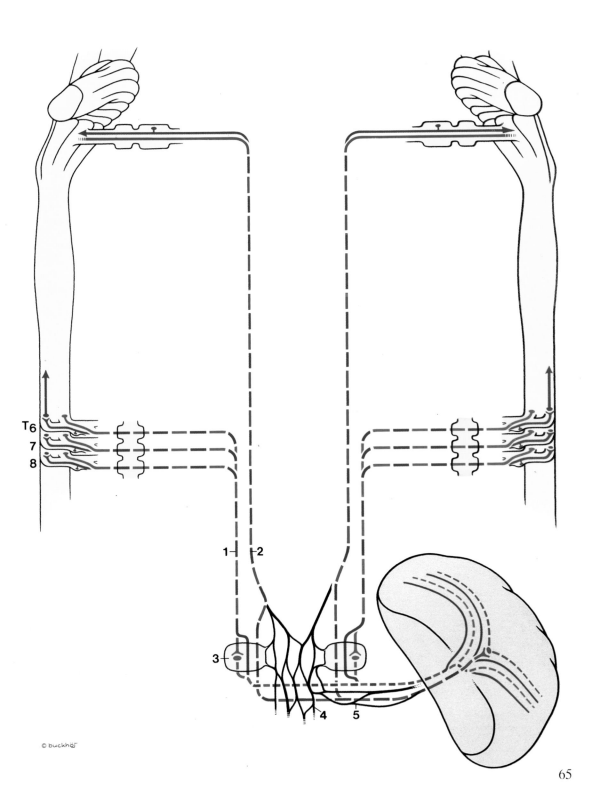

Small intestine

The small intestine, like most of the abdominal viscera, has sympathetic and vagal innervations. The sympathetic efferent fibers originate from the sixth to twelfth thoracic dermatomes and pass through the paravertebral sympathetic ganglia and via the splanchnic nerves to the celiac ganglion where they end. Postganglionic fibers reach the duodenum by way of the hepatic plexus and the jejunum and ileum through the superior mesenteric plexus. Afferent fibers, via the celiac plexus and splanchnic nerves, enter the spinal cord at the T9 – L1 levels.

The parasympathetic efferent innervation is primarily from the right vagus nerve. Afferent innervation starts in the end-organ and passes through the celiac plexus to ascend in the vagal trunks.

Fig. 1.51. Innervation of the small intestine.

Afferent fibers
——————— Vagal, parasympathetic
——————— Sympathetic

Efferent fibers
——————— Vagal, parasympathetic preganglionic
.— — — — — Vagal, parasympathetic postganglionic
——————— Sympathetic, preganglionic
.— — — — — Sympathetic, postganglionic

1. Vagus nerve
2. Anterior esophageal branches
3. Posterior esophageal branches
4. Celiac plexus
5. Greater splanchnic nerve
6. Lesser splanchnic nerve
7. Least splanchnic nerve
8. Celiac ganglion
9. Aorticorenal ganglion
10. Superior mesenteric plexus
11. Superior mesenteric ganglion
12. Plexus surrounding gastroduodenal artery
13. Duodenum
14. Jejunum
15. Ileum

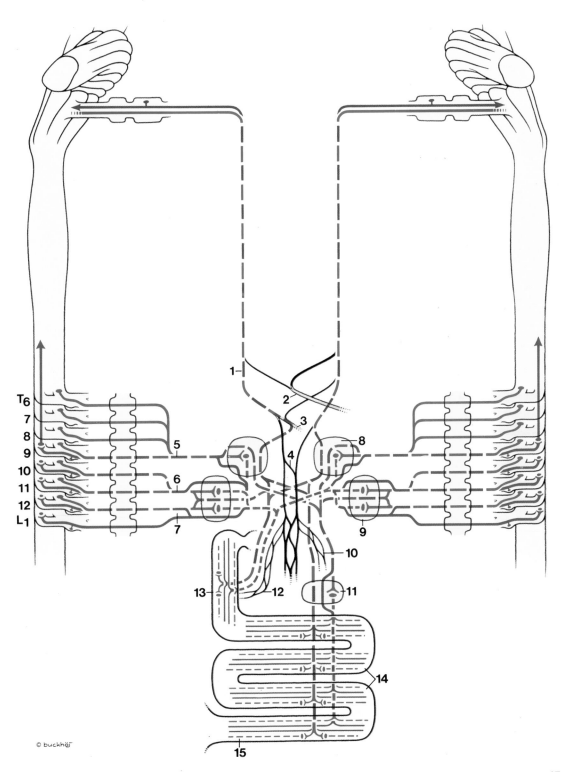

T6
7
8
9
10
11
12
L1

1–
2
3
5
4
8
6
9
7
10
11
13– 12
14
15

© buckhöj

Appendix

The appendix sympathetic efferent innervation originates at T11 and T12. These preganglionic neurons pass via the splanchnic nerves to the celiac plexus. Postganglionic neurons from the celiac plexus follow the vasculature, by way of the superior mesenteric plexus, to terminate in the musculature of the appendix. Afferent innervation returns to the spinal cord following the same pathway. Parasympathetic innervation (efferent and afferent) is primarily from the right vagus.

Fig. 1.52. Innervation of the appendix

Afferent fibers
—————— Vagal, parasympathetic
—————— Sympathetic

Efferent fibers
—————— Vagal, parasympathetic preganglionic
· — — — — Vagal, parasympathetic postganglionic
—————— Sympathetic, preganglionic
· — — — — Sympathetic, postganglionic

1. Vagus nerve
2. Lesser splanchnic nerve
3. Least splanchnic nerve
4. Celiac plexus
5. Celiac ganglion
6. Aorticorenal ganglion
7. Superior mesenteric ganglion
8. Superior mesenteric plexus

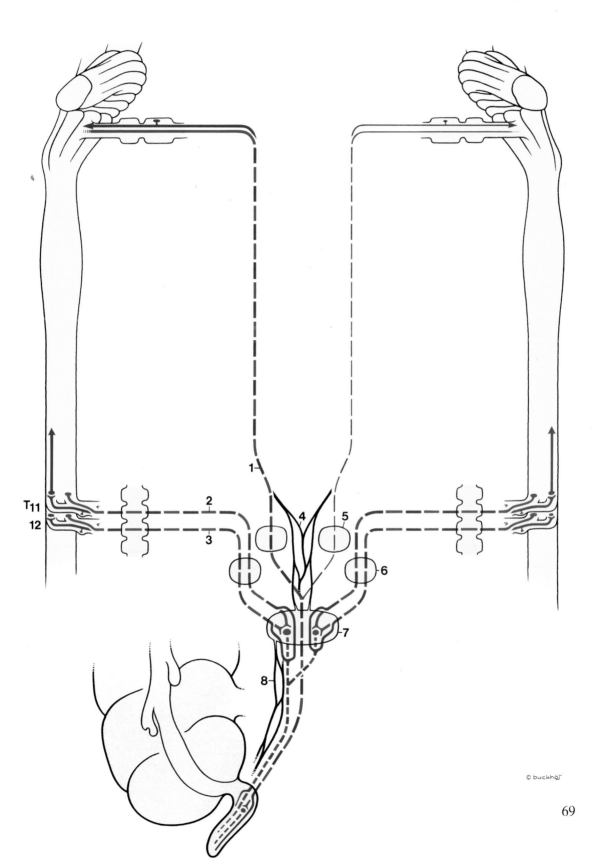

T$_{11}$

12

1

2

3

4

5

6

7

8

© buckhöj

69

Cecum and ascending and transverse colon

Sympathetic efferent innervation originates from T6 through T11. The nerves pass through the paravertebral ganglia to the celiac ganglia. Postganglionic fibers follow the arterial system, via the superior mesenteric plexus, to the musculature of the large intestine. Afferent branches return to the cord following the same pathways, ending at T9 – L1.

Parasympathetic efferent innervation is by way of both vagus nerves although primarily the right vagus is involved. Afferent innervation starts in the end-organ and returns via the celiac plexus to the vagal trunks.

Fig. 1.53. Innervation of the cecum and the ascending and transverse colon.

Afferent fibers
——— Vagal, parasympathetic
——— Sympathetic

Efferent fibers
——— Vagal, parasympathetic preganglionic
·— — — Vagal, parasympathetic postganglionic
——— Sympathetic, preganglionic
·— — — Sympathetic, postganglionic

1. Vagus nerve
2. Greater splanchnic nerve
3. Lesser splanchnic nerve
4. Least splanchnic nerve
5. First lumbar splanchnic nerve
6. Celiac plexus
7. Celiac ganglion
8. Aorticorenal ganglion
9. Superior mesenteric ganglion
10. Superior mesenteric plexus
11. Cecum
12. Ascending colon
13. Transverse colon

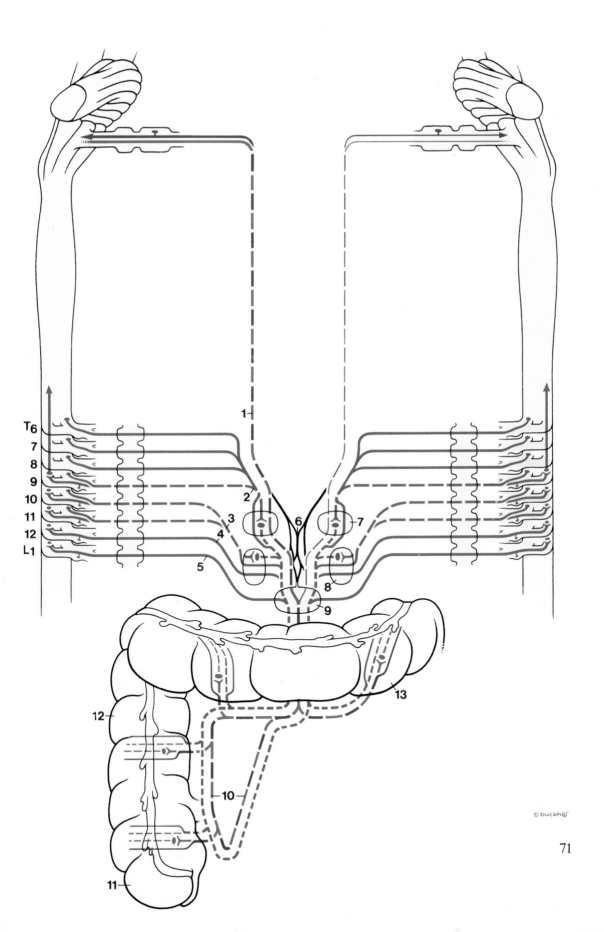

Descending colon, sigmoid colon and rectum

Sympathetic efferent fibers arise in the lower portion of the cord and pass through the upper lumbar sympathetic ganglia and aortic plexus to the inferior mesenteric plexus. Postganglionic fibers then follow the vessels to the distal colon. In addition some sympathetic fibers go to the rectum via the pelvic plexus.

The afferent sympathetic innervation is as follows: from the descending colon to the sigmoid afferent supply enters the cord at the T9 – T12 level on the left; from the sigmoid fibers pass to T11 – L1, also on the left.

Parasympathetic efferent innervation is primarily through the second, third, and fourth sacral nerves via the pelvic plexus.

These fibers have been given the name of nervi erigentes. It is possible that some parts of the distal colon also receive parasympathetic fibers from the vagus. The anus and external anal sphincter also receive innervation from the inferior hemorrhoidal branch of the pudendal nerve. Afferent parasympathetic innervation is via S2, 3 and 4.

Sphincter control is chiefly dependent on intact function of the S3 root.

Fig. 1.54. Innervation of the descending colon, sigmoid, and rectum.

Afferent fibers
———— Parasympathetic
———— Sympathetic
———— Parasympathetic (19)

Efferent fibers
———— Vagal, parasympathetic preganglionic
·----- Vagal, parasympathetic postganglionic
———— Sympathetic, preganglionic
·----- Sympathetic, postganglionic
———— Parasympathetic, preganglionic (18)
·----- Parasympathetic, postganglionic (18)
———— Parasympathetic, preganglionic (19)
·----- Parasympathetic, postganglionic (19)

1. Vagus nerve
2. Greater splanchnic nerve
3. Lesser splanchnic nerve
4. Least splanchnic nerve
5. Lumbar splanchnic nerve
6. Celiac ganglion
7. Aorticorenal ganglion
8. Superior mesenteric ganglion
9. Inferior mesenteric ganglion
10. Superior hypogastric plexus
11. Inferior mesenteric plexus
12. Pelvic plexus
13. Descending colon
14. Sigmoid colon
15. Rectum
16. Anus
17. Pelvic ganglion
18. Pelvic splanchnic nerves
    (nervi erigentes)
19. Pudendal nerve

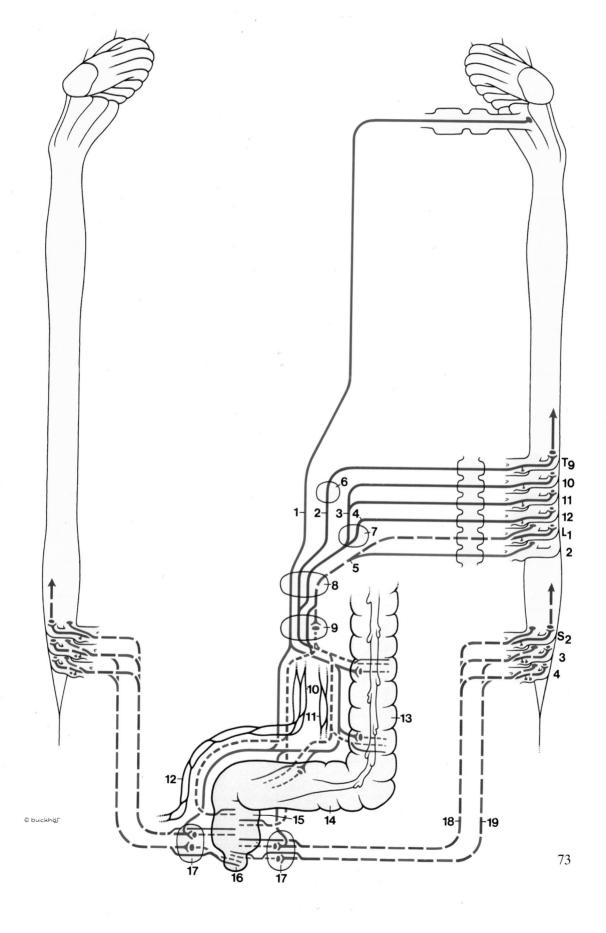

T9
10
11
12
L1
2

6

1 2 3 4

7

5

8

9

10

11

13

12

15 14

18 19

17

16

17

S2
3
4

© buckhöj

73

Kidney and ureter

The origin of the sympathetic efferent innervation is T10 – T12 and L1. Postganglionic fibers from the celiac plexus, aortic plexus and upper lumbar sympathetic chain run to the kidney and the upper part of the ureter. The lower part of the ureter is supplied by way of the superior and inferior hypogastric plexuses. Afferent innervation returns to spinal cord levels T10 – L1.

Efferent parasympathetic innervation for the kidney and the upper part of the ureter consists of vagal fibers passing through the celiac plexus for the most part. However, some vagal fibers join the renal plexus directly. The middle and lower parts of the ureter receive sacral parasympathetic innervation from S2 to S4.

Fig. 1.55. Innervation of the kidneys and ureters.

Afferent fibers
Parasympathetic
Sympathetic

Efferent fibers
Vagal, parasympathetic preganglionic
Vagal, parasympathetic postganglionic
Sympathetic, preganglionic
Sympathetic, postganglionic
Parasympathetic, preganglionic (11)
Parasympathetic, postganglionic (11)

1. Lumbar splanchnic nerve
2. Least splanchnic nerve
3. Lesser splanchnic nerve
4. Vagus nerve
5. Celiac ganglion
6. Superior mesenteric ganglion
7. Renal ganglion
8. Renal plexus
9. Superior hypogastric plexus
10. Inferior hypogastric plexus
11. Pelvic splanchnic nerves
    (nervi erigentes)

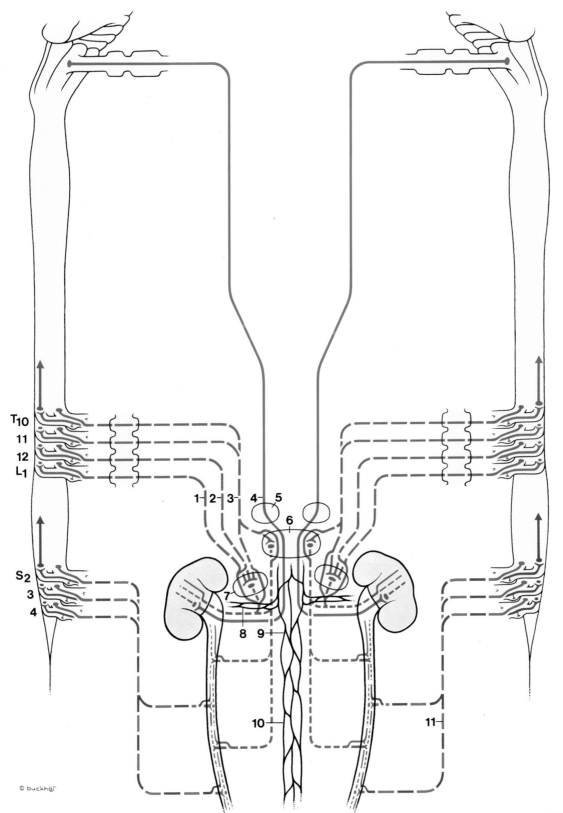

© buckhöj

75

Bladder and urethra

Sympathetic efferent innervation is from the lower thoracic dermatomes and L1. These preganglionic fibers pass directly through the lumbar and aortic plexus to the superior hypogastric plexus. Hypogastric postganglionic twigs go via the pelvic plexus to the body of the bladder. Sympathetic afferent innervation is primarily to T11, T12, and L1. The trigone and neck of the bladder receive their motor and sensory innervation from the second, third and fourth sacral nerves.

Intact sphincter function is chiefly dependent on S3 .

Fig. 1.56. Innervation of the bladder and urethra.

Afferent fibers
———— Parasympathetic
———— Sympathetic

Efferent fibers
———— Sympathetic, preganglionic
·————— Sympathetic, postganglionic
———— Parasympathetic, preganglionic
·————— Parasympathetic, postganglionic

1. Lesser splanchnic nerve
2. Least splanchnic nerve
3. Lumbar splanchnic nerve
4. Celiac ganglion
5. Aorticorenal ganglion
6. Inferior mesenteric ganglion
7. Hypogastric plexus
8. Pelvic splanchnic nerves (nervi erigentes)
9. Pelvic plexus
10. Trigone
11. Pelvic ganglion

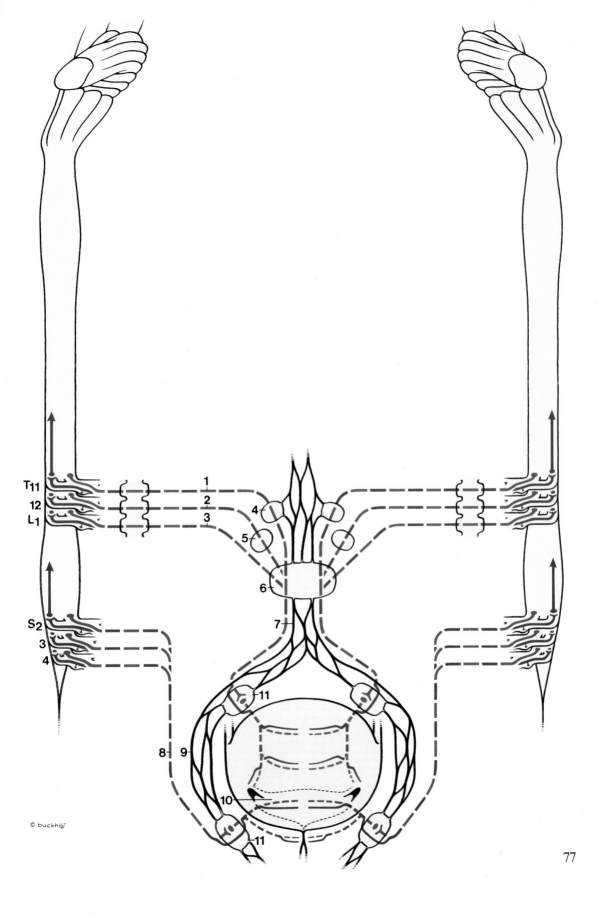

T11

12

L1

S2

3

4

1
2
3

4

5

6

7

8 9

10

11

11

© buckhöj

77

Uterus

Sympathetic preganglionic efferents have their origin from T5 to the lumbar end of the spinal cord. Some fibers pass, as part of the splanchnic nerves, through the celiac, aortic, inferior mesenteric and superior hypogastric plexuses, to the pelvic plexus. Other preganglionic fibers synapse in the celiac, aortic, paravertebral, and prevertebral ganglia. Postganglionic fibers follow the vascular supply to the uterus and related structures.

Parasympathetic preganglionic efferent innervation is from the S2 – S4 fibers which, via the nervi erigentes or pelvic splanchnic nerves, reach the myometrium. Postganglionic fibers start in the organ and supply it and adjacent tissues (i.e., fallopian tubes, etc.).

Sympathetic afferents return to the cord from the body of the uterus via T10 – L1, primarily T11 and T12. Parasympathetic afferents from the cervix return via S2 – S4.

Fig. 1.57. Innervation of the uterus.

Afferent fibers
—————— Parasympathetic
—————— Sympathetic

Efferent fibers
—————— Sympathetic, preganglionic
·— — — — Sympathetic, postganglionic
—————— Parasympathetic, preganglionic
·— — — — Parasympathetic, postganglionic

1. Greater splanchnic nerve
2. Lesser splanchnic nerve
3. Least splanchnic nerve
4. Lumbar splanchnic nerve
5. Celiac plexus
6. Celiac ganglion
7. Aorticorenal ganglion
8. Superior mesenteric ganglion
9. Ovarian plexus
10. Aorticoabdominal plexus
11. Inferior mesenteric ganglion
12. Superior and inferior hypogastric plexuses
13. Pelvic ganglion
14. Pelvic plexus
15. Pelvic splanchnic nerves (nervi erigentes)

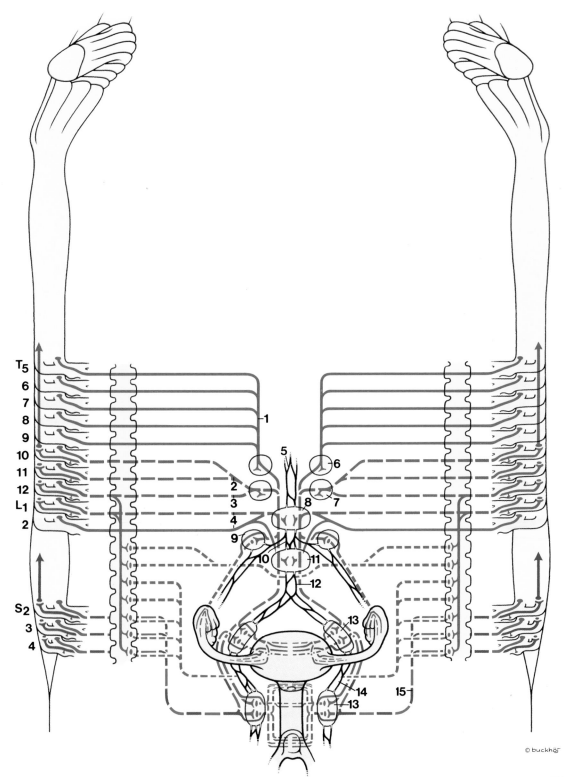

T5
6
7
8
9
10
11
12
L1
2

1

5
6
2
3
8
7
4
9
10
11
12
13
14
13
15

S2
3
4

© buckhöj

79

2. Block techniques

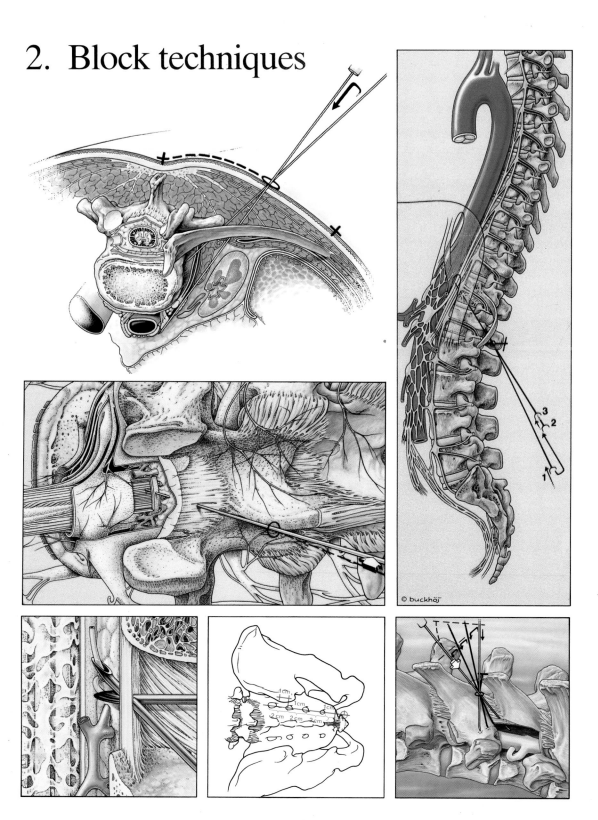

© buckhöj

81

Introduction

Preparation of patient

When performing a regional anesthetic the patient should be adequately informed about the block procedure to be undertaken. This is far more useful than any type of pharmacologic premedication.

In some cases, especially when the block is a painful one, narcotic premedication might be needed. For lesser block procedures sedating or tranquilizing agents are indicated. Rarely should anticholinergic drugs be used since the drying and vagolytic effects are not needed. A favorite form of premedication is diazepam, 0.1 – 0.2 mg/kg by mouth, which in addition to its tranquilizing effects also elevates the seizure threshold, thus protecting the patient slightly against the potential CNS toxicity effects of the local anesthetics.

Contraindications

The general contraindications to regional anesthesia consist of significant coagulation disorders, known allergy to local anesthetics, infection at the site of injection and, for spinal and epidural anesthesia, certain neurologic diseases and hypovolemia. There are also some relative contraindications such as anatomic aberrations – congenital or acquired – which will render the regional anesthetic procedure difficult or the result unpredictable.

Consent

The patient's consent should always be obtained after proper information has been presented, not only about the advantages but also about the potential risks. This is particularly important before neurolytic procedures. It should not be permitted for a patient who was promised general anesthesia to be talked into regional anesthesia after he has been premedicated unless the reasons are extremely cogent and appropriate administrative concurrence has been obtained. Documentation of the reasons for the change should be adequately detailed in the patient's medical records.

Safety precautions

For any regional anesthetic procedure equipment and drugs for resuscitation should always be available. The following is a list of the minimum needed when a major block is to be performed:

1. An intravenous needle in place

2. Equipment for positive pressure ventilation
   a) oxygen
   b) equipment for endotracheal intubation
   c) self-inflating bag and mask

3. Drugs
   a) diazepam or midazolam
   b) thiopental and succinylcholine
   c) a syringe prefilled with a vasopressor agent such as ephedrine, 10 mg/ml
   d) colloid or crystalloid fluids

Procedure

The procedure should be carried out as expeditiously and gently as possible while reassuring the patient and informing him of what is to be expected next in the technique. Infiltration of the soft tissues with generous amounts of dilute local anesthetic solutions injected with minimal pressure, use of as fine a block needle as possible, and the deliberate movement of the needle all contribute to an optimal technique. Such seemingly minor details make nerve block anesthesia a more acceptable method to patients, surgeons, and other medical personnel involved in the care of the patient.

As a general rule blocks should not be performed in anesthetized patients as inadvertent neural puncture or intraneural injections cannot be detected. In addition the quality and distribution of the block cannot be evaluated so the block will more or less be a "shot in the dark."

After the technique is completed the anesthesiologist must determine the adequacy of the block for surgery. If necessary, appropriate supplementation prior to the start of surgery, repetition of the block, or use of a light general anesthetic might be required to augment a partially effective regional anesthetic technique.

Verification of correct placement of the needle

In order to minimize the failure rate of blocks great care should be taken to obtain optimal positioning of the needle tip. Anatomic landmarks, as described for the various block procedures, are in most cases sufficient. For some blocks additional measures should be taken:

1. Elicitation of paresthesias. Sensory paresthesias indicate that the nerve has been hit by the tip of the needle and more or less guarantees optimal needle placement. Under no circumstance should the injection of local anesthetics be continued if the initial part of the injection is accompanied by severe paresthesias.

2. X-ray verification. The correct positioning of the needle tip in relation to bony structures can be verified by roentgenograms or, preferably, fluoroscopy in two planes. In the upper thoracic area this method is of limited value. By noticing the spread of small amounts of a radio-opaque agent a further aid in the correct positioning of the needle can be obtained. The details are described below for some blocks. Anaphylactic reactions to radio-opaque agents sometimes occur and full resuscitative facilities should be at hand.

3. Nerve stimulators. A nerve stimulator is an excellent adjunct for the performance of some peripheral nerve blocks, especially in patients with difficult anatomy. In the thoraco-abdominal region they are seldom of importance. The basic principle of a nerve stimulator is to transmit an impulse which, when in the vicinity of a nerve, will cause an evoked response to occur. If the nerve is a motor or a mixed sensory – motor one, the evoked response will be in the form of a muscle twitch. By producing a maximal evoked response at a minimal current (0.5 – 1 mA), the proximity of the needle tip to the nerve is assured. Injection of 2 ml of a local anesthetic agent will abolish the evoked response as an indication of optimal needle position. Injection of the full dose of the local anesthetic or the neurolytic agent will almost always produce the desired block. For obvious reasons nerve stimulators cannot be used for the identification of autonomic nervous structures.

The authors prefer the use of sheathed needle electrodes to locate specific nerves. However, there are indications in the literature that ordinary needles made of conducting substances may work just as well.

Suggested reading

Bashein G, Haschke RH, Ready LB (1984) Electrical nerve location: numerical and electrophoretic comparison of insulated vs uninsulated needles. Anesth Analg 63:919

Ferrer-Brechner T, Brechner VL (1976) Accuracy of needle placement during diagnostic and therapeutic nerve blocks. In Bonica JJ, Albe-Fessard D (eds) Advances in pain research and therapy, vol 1, Raven Press, New York, p 679

Ford DJ, Pither C, Raj PP (1984) Comparison of insulated and uninsulated needles for locating peripheral nerves with a peripheral nerve stimulator. Anesth Analg 63:925

Goldberg M (1984) Systemic reactions to intravascular contrast media. A guide for the anesthesiologist. Anesthesiology 60:46

Hymes JA (1985) A simple, inexpensive needle assembly for peripheral nerve stimulation and neural blockade. Reg Anesth 10:197

Johans TG, Carr G (1985) Peripheral nerve stimulation through a local anesthetic path: a modified Koons technique. Anesth Analg 64:1217

Montgomery SJ, Raj PP, Nettles D et al (1973) The use of the nerve stimulator with standard unsheated needles in nerve blockade. Anesth Analg 52:827

Mylrea KC, Hameroff DR, Calkins JM et al (1984) Evaluation of peripheral nerve stimulators and relationship to possible errors in assessing neuromuscular blockade. Anesthesiology 60:464

Pither CE, Raj PP, Ford DJ (1985) The use of peripheral nerve stimulators for regional anesthesia. A review of experimental characteristics, technique and clinical applications. Reg Anaesth 10:49

Selander D, Dhunèr K-G, Lundborg G (1977) Peripheral nerve injury due to injection needles used for regional anaesthesia. An experimental study of the acute effects of needle point trauma. Acta Anaesthesiol Scand 21:182

Selander D, Edshage S, Wolff T (1979) Paraesthesia or no paraesthesia? Nerve lesions after axillary blocks. Acta Anaesthesiol Scand 23:27.

Selander D, Brattsand R, Lundborg G et al. (1979) Local anaesthetics: importance of mode of application, concentration and adrenaline for the appearance of nerve lesions. Acta Anaesthesiol Scand 23:127

Smith BL (1976) Efficacy of a nerve stimulator in regional analgesia: experience in a resident training programme. Anaesthesia 31:778

Local anesthetics

Although it is beyond the scope of this book to go into a definitive presentation of the properties of the various local anesthetics, some general statements should be made. There are many different local anesthetics, each available in a variety of concentrations with or without the addition of adrenaline. This wide selection permits a high degree of individualization as to the onset, duration, and intensity of the block.

The local anesthetics are classified either as shortacting, such as lidocaine, prilocaine, and mepivacaine, or longacting such as tetracaine, bupivacaine, and etidocaine. Their duration of action varies widely with the type of block performed but is approximately 2 h for the shortacting and 8 – 12 h for the longacting agents when administered to peripheral nerves.

The properties of the shortacting local anesthetics do not differ to any major extent, with the exception of significantly lower toxicity with prilocaine. On the other hand this agent may cause methemoglobinemia.

Of the longacting agents bupivacaine has a comparatively long onset time whereas etidocaine, which has a short onset time, causes profound motor blockade that can cause the clinically unwanted situation of returning sensation in a nonmobile extremity. Tetracaine is used primarily for spinals.

By employing various concentrations of an agent a differential nerve block is achieved to some extent. For example, lidocaine 0.5%, 1.0% and 2.0% results primarily in sympathetic, sympathetic and sensory, and sympathetic, sensory and motor block, respectively. This delineation, however, is not as precise as we once thought.

In general, as dilute a solution as possible should be used in order to reduce the risk of toxicity, i.e., for the shortacting agents

0.25% – 0.5% solution for infiltration anesthesia, 1% for peripheral nerve blocks, and 2% for epidural anesthesia. Usually, adrenaline-containing solutions should be used since they result in lower plasma concentrations and more profound blocks of longer duration than do plain solutions. There are certain areas of the body, such as the digits or penis, where adrenaline-containing solutions should never be used since the vasoconstriction caused may lead to tissue necrosis.

For each drug there exists a maximal dose that should not be exceeded. It must be remembered that patient related factors will often reduce the maximal dose which may be used. Renal, hepatic and cardiac diseases, dehydration, malnutrition and acidosis are examples of conditions that reduce the maximal amount of local anesthetic which should be given. In addition, the systemic uptake of a local anesthetic varies considerably between different regions of the body as well as between areas in which nerve blocks are done. For example, absorption from head and neck structures is much greater than from the soft tissue of the back. Similarly, it is known that blood levels after intercostal blocks are much higher than those when the same amount of local anesthetic is used for other peripheral nerve blocks.

The following table provides general guidelines to the maximum doses (mg/kg body weight) of various agents:

Table 1. General guidelines to the maximum doses (mg/kg body weight) of various agents.

Agent	plain	with adrenaline
Lidocaine	5	7
Mepivacaine	5	5
Prilocaine	7	9
Bupivacaine	2–3	2–3
Etidocaine	4	5

Prior to any injection of a local anesthetic it should be ascertained that the needle tip is not intravascular since a rapid rise in blood levels secondary to inadvertent intravascular injection is the prime cause of toxic reactions. Repeated aspirations should be carried out during the performance of any nerve block procedure. This becomes of critical importance when injections are done next to arterial systems going directly to the brain, i.e., for a stellate ganglion block, where injection into the vertebral artery is a rare but potential complication. Even a few milligrams of any local anesthetic injected directly into the cerebral circulation could cause a grand-mal convulsion.

In general toxic symptoms progress in a typical order. They start with minor central nervous system manifestations, e.g., dizziness, ringing in the ears, sensation of lightheadedness, and metallic taste in the mouth. This can progress to skeletal muscle twitching and nystagmus, which may be followed by generalized convulsive movements. Ordinarily cardiovascular collapse will not occur unless the circulating plasma concentrations of local anesthetic are extremely high or the acidosis, increased oxygen demand, decreased ventilation causing hypoxia, etc. secondary to the convulsion are not adequately treated. The compounding of these effects by the high local anesthetic levels can cause cardiac arrest.

The treatment of mild CNS toxic effects should consist of oxygenation plus either diazepam 0.1 – 0.2 mg/kg or 25 – 50 mg thiopental (Pentothal) intravenously. If frank convulsions occur, thiopental or succinylcholine together with artificial ventilation should be given immediately. The earlier the recognition of the symptoms of toxicity the better the chance of not allowing them to proceed to frank convulsions or cardiovascular collapse. It is therefore imperative that the anesthesiologist keep in contact verbally with the patient throughout the technical performance of the block and immediately postblock. Overly heavy sedation or general anesthesia is contraindicated.

Anaphylactic reactions to local anesthetics of the amide type are extremely rare. They are not dosedependent and may occur even after injection of minor amounts. Treatment is that of anaphylactic reactions in general. It is of great importance to both the patient and his doctor to clarify whether the patient has an allergy to local anesthetics. Analysis of the patient's history and any earlier complications resulting from regional anesthesia may be sufficient to rule out differential diagnoses such as vasovagal syncope or reaction to adrenaline, but an additional allergy workup should be undertaken in the suspect case. If the patient actually is allergic he should be provided with a written statement by the investigating physician.

Suggested reading

Albright GA (1979) Cardiac arrest following regional anesthesia with etidocaine or bupivacaine. Anesthesiology 51:285

Aldrete JA, Johnson DA (1970) Evaluation of intracutaneous testing for investigation of allergy to local anesthetic agents. Anesth Analg 49:173

Aldrete JA, Usubiaga LE (1979) New concepts of toxicity for local anesthetic agents. Reg Anaesth 4:6

Brown DT, Beamish D, Wildsmith JAW (1981) Allergic reaction to an amide local anaesthetic. Br J Anaesth 53:435

Clarkson CW, Hondeghem L, Matsubara T et al (1984) Possible mechanism of bupivacaine toxicity: fast inactivation block with slow diastolic recovery (abstract). Anesth Analg 63:199

Cotton BR, Henderson HP, Achola KJ et al (1986) Changes in plasma catecholamine concentrations following infiltration with large volumes of local anaesthetic solution containing adrenaline. Br J Anaesth 58:593

Covino BG, Vasallo H (1976) Local anesthetics. Mechanism of action and clinical use. In: Kitz RJ, Laver MB (eds) The scientific basis of clinical anesthesia. Grune & Stratton, New York.

Covino BG (1986) Pharmacology of local anaesthetic agents. Br J Anaest 58:701

Edde RR, Deutsch S (1977) Cardiac arrest efter interscalene brachial plexus block. Anesth Analg 56:446

Fisher MMcD, Pennington JC (1982) Allergy to local anaesthesia. Br J Anaesth 54:893

Ford DJ, Raj PP, Sing P et al. (1984) Differential peripheral nerve block by local anesthetics in the cat. Anesthesiology 60:28

Incaudo G, Schatz M, Patterson R et al.(1978) Administration of local anesthetics to patients with a history of prior adverse reaction. J Allergy Clin Immunol 61:339

Kasten GW, Martin ST (1984) Successful resuscitation after massive intravenous bupivacaine overdose in hypoxic dog. Anesthesiology 61:A206

Kotelko DM, Shnider SM, Brizgys RV et al. (1984) Bupivacaine induced arrhythmias in sheep. Anesthesiology 60:10

Marx GF (1984) Cardiotoxicity of local anesthetics – the plot thickens. Anesthesiology 60:3

Mather EM, Cousins MJ (1979) Local anaesthetics and their current clinical use. Drugs 18:185

Moore DC, Crawford RD, Scurlock JE (1980) Severe hypoxia and acidosis following local anesthetic-induced convulsions. Anesthesiology 53:259

Prentiss JE (1979) Cardiac arrest following caudal anesthesia. Anesthesiology 50:51

Reiz S, Nath S (1986) Cardiotoxicity of local anaesthetic agents. Br J Anaesth 58:736

Rosen MA, Thigpen JW, Shnider SM et al. (1985) Bupivacaine-induced cardiotoxicity in hypoxic and acidotic sheep. Anesth Analg 64:1089

Scott DB (1975) Evaluation of the toxicity of local anaesthetic agents in man. Br J Anaesth 47:56

Scott DB (1986) Toxicity effects of local anaesthetic agents on the central nervous system. Br J Anaesth 58:732

Strichartz G (1978) Molecular mechanisms of nerve block by local anesthetics. Anesthesiology 45:421

Thigpen JW, Kotelko DM, Shnider SM et al. (1983) Bupivacaine cardiotoxicity in hypoxic-acidotic sheep. Anesthesiology 59:A204

Thomas RD, Behbehani MM, Coyle DE et al (1986) Cardiovascular toxicity of local anesthetics: an alternative hypothesis. Anesth Analg 65:444

Tucker GT, Mather LE (1979) Clinical pharmacokinetics of local anaesthetics. Clin Pharmacokinet 4:241

Tucker GT (1986) Pharmacokinetics of local anaesthetics. Br J Anaesth 58:717

Wiklund L (1984) Cardiovascular and central nervous system toxicity of local anaesthetics. Ann Chir Gynaecol 73:123

Wildsmith JAW (1985) Prilocaine – an underused local anesthetic. Reg Anaesth 10:155

Wildsmith JAW (1986) Peripheral nerve and local anaesthetic drugs. Br J Anaesth 58:692

Wojtczak JA, Griffin RM, Pratilas V et al. (1984) Is it possible to resuscitate a bupivacaine-intoxicated heart? Anesthesiology 61:A207

Writer WDR, Davis JM, Strunin L (1984) Trial by media: the bupivacaine story. Can Anaesth Soc J 31:1

In cases where block procedures are used for prolonged pain relief, one has to resort to either repetitive blocks, continuous techniques, narcotics, or, occasionally, neurolytic blocks with alcohol or phenol.

Narcotics

Within the last few years the use of epidural and intrathecal narcotics for the management of a variety of painful situations has been reintroduced into medicine. Although tests have shown many of the available narcotics to provide analgesia, those primarily used at the time of writing are morphine and fentanyl. There are advantages and disadvantages to each of these agents.

Morphine, which is a more polar compound, when given in the epidural or intrathecal space tends to have a prolonged action – anywhere from 8 to 24 h after a single injection. The onset time is 30 – 60 min. Fentanyl, a much more highly lipid soluble agent, has a duration of action which is usually considered to be 3 – 6 h after an onset time of 10 – 20 min.

Morphine produces the unwanted effects of itching, urinary retention, and occasionally respiratory depression. Potentially life-threatening respiratory depression may be seen many hours after the initial injection of morphine. The usual reason presented for this is that morphine, due to its higher polarity, is not as easily bound to the lipid components of the spinal cord. Hence, some of the morphine molecules will be freefloating in the CSF, eventually rising to bathe the respiratory centers in the medulla, thus causing depression. Although all of the mentioned unwanted effects of morphine do occur with fentanyl, they do so with a far lower incidence. In fact, respiratory depression after fentanyl is an extremely rare event. This is due to the fact that fentanyl, being more lipid soluble, remains more firmly attached to spinal cord lipoproteins.

Intrathecal morphine is usually given in doses of 0.5 – 1.0 mg. Published papers report a range between 0.03 and 20 (sic!) mg. A high incidence of delayed respiratory depression with the use of intrathecal morphine has been reported. Epidurally, doses of 2 – 8 mg may be used. The epidural fentanyl dose is ordinarily 0.1 mg.

Spinal opiate analgesia has not yet become the panacea that early reports appeared to promise. Many questions remain unanswered, but the concept on which this modality of pain treatment was based has been declared one of the most important recent developments in medicine.

Suggested reading

Bromage PR, Camporesi EM, Durant PACV et al. (1982) Nonrespiratory side effects of epidural morphine. Anesth Analg 61:490

Corke CF, Wheatley RG (1985) Respiratory depression complicating epidural diamorphine. Two case reports of administration after dural puncture. Anaesthesia 40:1203

Dahlström B (1986) Pharmacokinetics and pharmacodynamics of epidural and intrathecal morphine. Int Anesthesiol Clin 24:29

Cousins MJ, Mather EM (1984) Intrathecal and epidural administration of opioids. Anesthesiology 61:276

Donadini R, Rolly G, Noorduin H et al. (1985) Epidural sufentanil for postoperative pain relief. Anaesthesia 40:634

Glynn CJ, Mather LE, Cousins MJ et al (1981) Peridural meperidine in humans. Analgetic response, pharmacokinetics, and transmission into CSF. Anesthesiology 55:520

Gourlay GK, Cherry DA, Cousins MJ (1985) Cephalad migration of morphine in CSF following lumbar epidural administration in patients with cancer pain. Pain 23:317

Gustafsson LL, Grell AM, Gark M et al. (1984) Kinetics of morphine in cerebrospinal fluid after epidural administration. Acta Anaesth Scand 28:535

Gustafsson LL, Post C, Edvardsen et al. (1985) Distribution of morphine and meperidine after intrathecal administration in rat and mouse. Anesthesiology 63:483

Jacobson L (1984) Intrathecal and extradural narcotics. In: Benedetti C et al (eds) Advances in pain research and therapy, vol 7. Raven Press, New York, p 199

Korbon GA, James DJ, Verlander JM et al. (1985) Intramuscular naloxone reverses the side effects of epidural morphine while preserving analgesia. Reg Anaesth 10:16

Magora F, Cotev S (1986) Future trends in regional spinal opioids. Int Anaesthesiol Clin 24:113

Moore RA, Bullingham RES, McQuay HJ et al. (1982) Dural permeability to narcotics: in vitro determination and application to extradural administration. Br J Anaesth 54:1117

Nordberg G (1984) Pharmacokinetic aspects of spinal morphine analgesia. Acta Anaesthesiol Scand 28 (suppl 79)

Nordberg G (1986) Epidural versus intrathecal route of opioid administration. Int Anaesthesiol Clin 24:93

Rawal N, Schött U, Dahlström B et al (1986) Influence of naloxone infusion on analgesia and respiratory depression following epidural morphine. Anesthesiology 64:194

Torda TA, Pybus DA (1984) Extradural administration of morphine and bupivacaine. A controlled comparison. Br J Anaesth 56:141

Yaksh TL (1981) Spinal opiate analgesia: characteristics and principles of action. Pain 11:293

Yaksh TL (1984) Multiple opioid receptor systems in brain and spinal cord: part 2. Eur J Anaesth 1:201

Yaksh T (1985) Pharmacology of spinal adrenergic systems which modulate spinal nociceptive processing. Pharmacol Biochem Behav 22:845

Neurolytic agents

For prolonged blocks, neurolytic agents may be indicated. The two most commonly used are alcohol and phenol.

Ethyl alcohol is an extremely potent neurolytic agent which acts on the neuron by the extraction of cholesterol, phospholipid and cerebroside. It causes precipitation of lipoproteins and aminoproteins. Concentrations of alcohol used clinically have varied from 50 to 100%. In our practice, when a neurolytic technique with alcohol is indicated (primarily for subarachnoid alcohol injection or the production of a chemical sympathectomy) 100% alcohol is the concentration chosen.

Phenol similarly causes protein denaturation. It is, like alcohol, extremely potent and nonselective in its neurodestructive abilities. Concentrations used vary from as little as 1% – 2% in sterile water for peripheral nerves in small children to 15% – 20% in hyperbaric solutions (i.e., dissolved in glycerine or similar substances) for subarachnoid injection in order to convert an adult spastic paraplegia to a flaccid one. Concentrations used to produce pain relief or chemical sympathectomy are commonly in the range of 5% – 10%.

The duration of effects one might see after a neurolytic block for either pain relief or sympathectomy varies considerably. This might be due to incomplete neurolysis or nerve regeneration. Most of the literature suggests that the effects of the block should generally last for 2–6 months. The authors, however, have seen blocks wear off within as short a time as 24 – 48 h. Conversely, occasionally a neurolytic injection will last for considerably longer than 6 months.

Indications for neurolytic blocks are limited and, in the context of the thoracoabdominal areas, primarily comprise subarachnoid injection for pain relief, chemical sympathectomy, or block of the celiac plexus. Owing to the complications associated with the use of these techniques, indications for the procedure must be definite in all cases.

It is strongly recommended that any neurolytic injection be preceded by a local anesthetic block for two reasons. First, one can determine the efficacy of the proposed procedure, i.e., to what extent the patient obtains pain relief. Secondly, and especially when blocks are performed to produce somatic analgesia, one occasionally finds that the resulting numbness is more distressing to the patient than his underlying painful condition.

The techniques for use of neurolytic blocks for subarachnoid injection, lumbar sympathectomy, and celiac plexus injection are described later. Except in unusual circumstances the authors do not advise the use of neurolytic agents for peripheral nerve blockade.

Suggested reading

Burkel WE, McPhee M (1970) Effect of phenol injection into peripheral nerve of the rat. Electron microscope studies. Arch Phys Med Rehabil 51:391

Felsenthal G (1974) Pharmacology of phenol in peripheral nerve block: a review. Arch Phys Med Rehabil 55:13

Fischer E, Cress RH, Haines G et al.(1970) Recovery of nerve conduction after nerve block by phenol. Am J Phys Med 50:230

Katz J, Joseph JW (1980) Neuropathology of neurolytic and semidestructive agents. In: Cousins MJ, Bridenbaugh PO,(eds) Neural blockade in clinical anesthesia and management of pain. J.B. Lippincott, Philadelphia, p 122.

Möller JE, Holweg-Larsen J, Jacobsen E (1969) Histopathological lesions in the sciatic nerve of the rat following perineural application of phenol and alcohol solution. Dan Med Bull 16:116

Smith MC (1964) Histological findings following intrathecal injection of phenol solutions for the relief of pain. Br J Anaesth 36:387

Wood KM (1978) The use of phenol as a neurolytic agent: review. Pain 5:205

Supplementary medication

Intraoperatively

Most patients are concerned with the anticipated discomfort of being awake during surgery. At the preoperative visit they should therefore be informed about the possibilities of obtaining a hypnotic agent while in the operating room. However, many patients prefer to stay awake once a personal relationship with the anesthesiologist has been established; they realize that they will "have a doctor of their own" concerned with their safety and well-being for the duration of the operation.

On the other hand, other patients absolutely demand to be asleep. Preferably this should be achieved with an intravenous agent that has a short elimination half-life. Various anesthesiologists have different preferences in this respect. A small intravenous dose of diazepam, 0.03 – 0.1 mg/kg, will usually provide some amnesia and sedation. Midazolam has a shorter half-life and is gaining popularity. For minute-to-minute control of the degree of sedation a continuous infusion of methohexitone can also be used.

The ventilatory or circulatory depressant effects of a combined regimen might become of significance when too profound sedation is accomplished.

Inhalation anesthesia by mask should only be necessary in children. Light general anesthesia concomitant with epidural anesthesia for major intra-abdominal procedures is described on p 157.

Occasionally the duration of surgery will prove to be longer than anticipated and exceed the duration of nerve block. For obvious reasons it is important to prevent any unnecessary suffering of the patient by providing additional analgesia or anesthesia. In some cases the surgeon can supplement the declining block by infiltration of a local anesthetic. In most cases, however, this is not possible. Administration of opioids parenterally usually yields unsatisfactory results or the opioids have to be administered in such high doses that respiratory depression ensues. In most cases it will suffice to infuse low-dose ketamine, approximately 0.5 – 1.0 ml of a 1 mg/ml solution per minute after an initial loading dose of 0.75 – 1.0 mg/kg body weight. With this small dose the patient might seem awake. In our experience ketamine administered in this way as an adjuvant to failing regional anesthesia has very few side-effects.

Suggested reading

Philip BK (1985) Supplemental medication of ambulatory procedures under regional anaesthesia. Anesth Analg 64:1117

Reves JG, Fragen RJ, Vinik R et al. (1985) Midazolam: pharmacology and uses. Anesthesiology 62:310

Postoperatively

Even if it is possible by regional anesthetic techniques to keep the patient pain free or almost pain free from the area of surgery, it is common for patients to complain of discomfort or pain from the throat, intravenous lines, oxygen masks, noise and smell in the recovery room, etc. Preferably the regional block should be supplemented by mild sedative and/or analgesic agents.

For evaluation or treatment of chronic pain

In order to make a correct assessment of the efficacy of any regional anesthetic procedure for the relief of chronic pain, pain medication should ideally be discontinued 6 – 8 h before the block. During the course of a continuous block or after a neurolytic block supplementary pain medication is an important component of the total care of the patient and should not be withheld. Records of the consumption of pain medication provide important information on the efficacy of the block and may constitute a basis for the decision on when and if the block should be repeated.

Records

For all regional anesthetic procedures a record should be kept not only of the type of block performed, but also how it was accomplished (including the anesthetic administered), whether any complications occurred, the nature of continued monitoring or treatment and how the patient responded to the procedure.

1. Type of block performed

In most countries there are various codes that denote the various anesthetic techniques. They are usually not specific enough to allow for a reasonably accurate description of the single or combined nerve blocking procedure that was actually performed. Therefore it is often necessary to describe this in words on the anesthesia chart.

2. Procedure

A brief description of the technique is sufficient. Of interest for retrospective reviews or one's own evaluation is to note whether paresthesias were elicited, whether a successful block resulted, the need for supplementation, any signs of complications and the patient's response to the procedure. It is mandatory to state the type and amount of local anesthetic given.

3. Complications

Records of vital signs should be kept for the duration of the block. For neurolytic procedures results of neurologic examinations of the patient performed prior to the block and at various stages after the block should be kept.

4. Written orders for the continued monitoring or treatment of the patient.

These could include top-up doses of local anesthetic or opioids for postoperative pain relief (agent, dose, interval), degree of ambulation of patient, etc in addition to conventional postoperative orders.

5. Follow-up of patient.

We consider it very important that a postoperative visit is made in order to find out how the patient experienced the regional anesthetic procedure and subsequent operation. Casual discussions with patients postoperatively is an important part of the anesthesiologist's visit to the wards. It is also very important to find out about any untoward sequelae of the nerve block and to institute appropriate remedial therapy. In contrast to general anesthesia, untoward sequelae, i.e., headache after spinal, often do not show up until many hours or even days after the procedure. It is therefore wise to ask the nurses in the wards or one's surgical colleagues to report any aberrations in late postoperative recovery, especially in patients who have undergone major regional anesthesia.

Lumbar spinal analgesia

Fig. 2.1. Spinal puncture by the midline approach at the L2 – L3 interspace. The spinal needle is in the midline directed slightly cephalad.

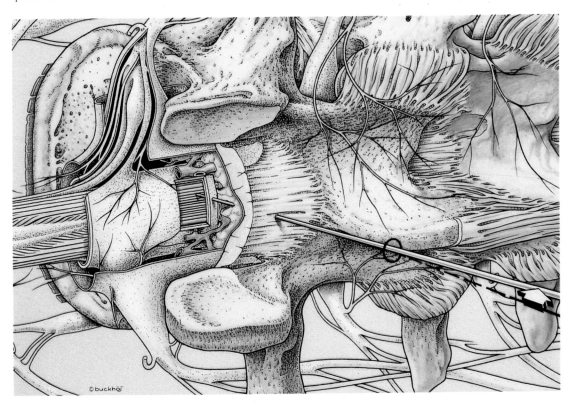

Single shot technique

Midline approach

The patient could be positioned either in a lateral position or in the sitting position (Fig. 2.2). For the patient's comfort the lateral position is generally to be preferred. For the less experienced anesthesiologist and in very obese patients the sitting position is recommended. If there is to be unilateral surgery, e.g., for an inguinal hernia, the side to be operated on should be downward. The patient's downward shoulder and his head are flexed toward the knees, and the head is supported on a pillow. An assistant is of great aid in helping the patient to assume and maintain this position.

The L2-L3 or L3-L4 interspace is identified by using a line between the iliac crests. This line will bisect the spinal process of the L4 vertebra. The spinal tap should be attempted at one of the above-mentioned interspaces. In more cranial interspaces there is always a risk of damaging the spinal cord, while at more caudad interspaces the distance from the skin is often greater, so that a spinal tap is comparatively more difficult to accomplish.

Fig. 2.2. Patient in the sitting position supported by the leg rests of a urologic operating table.

Fig. 2.3. Patient in the lateral position supported by an assistant.

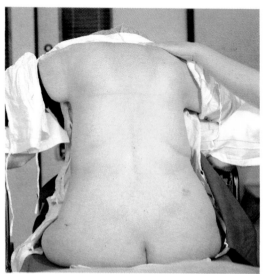

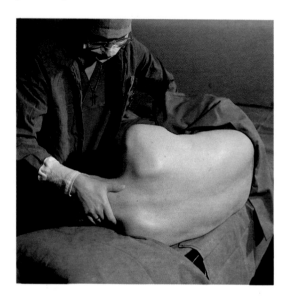

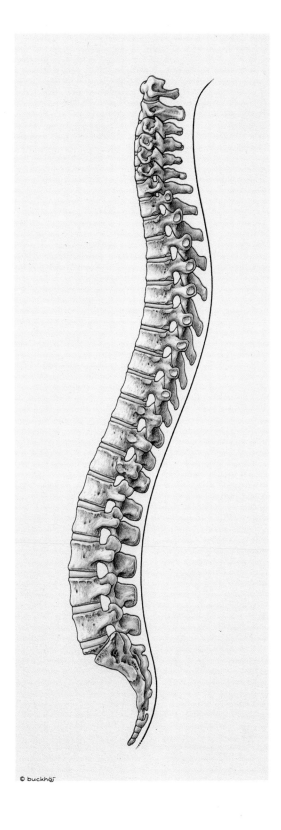

A 22-gauge, or preferably 25- or even 26-gauge, 10-cm spinal needle is used. In almost all cases spinal taps can be accomplished using a 25-gauge needle with or without an introducer.

The thumb of the left hand is placed on the inferior edge of the dorsal spine above the interspace to be punctured if the patient is in the left lateral position. In the right lateral position the thumb is placed below the interspace. The spinal needle is introduced through a skin wheal just below (above) the thumb. The needle, with the bevel in the longitudinal direction, is advanced slightly cephalad at an angle of 10° – 30° in the midline.

Fig. 2.4. The skin surface in relation to the spinous processes of the spinal column. Observe that the distance from the skin to the spinal canal is greater at the L5 – S1 intrespace than at L2 – L3.

Fig. 2.5. The path of the spinal needle through the supraspinous and interspinous ligaments.

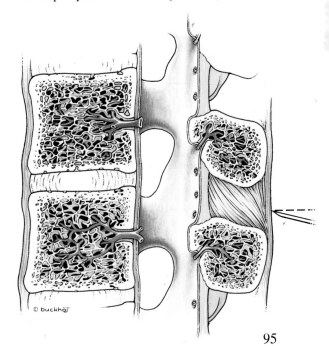

It is of great help to verify that the direction of the needle is correct by observing it from two vantage points (Fig. 2.6). The superficial portions of the interspinous ligament are identified by noting increased resistance once the needle passes through the subcutaneous tissue. The deeper layers of the interspinous ligament and the ligamentum flavum should be noted in the form of further increased resistance when the needle is advanced. The needle then enters the epidural space, which will be felt as a loss or decrease in resistance to advancement. At this point the stylet is removed to ascertain that there is no flow of CSF. The stylet is then replaced and the dura/arachnoid pierced slowly.

Free flowing, clear CSF should be noted in the hub of the needle, also after it has been rotated 90°. When employing the thin 25-gauge needle it is often very valuable to add a drop of the local anesthetic to the hub of the needle, which enables more rapid detection of a free flow of CNS through the needle.

Spinal puncture can sometimes be difficult. In most cases the difficulties reflect a faulty technique and not insurmountable anatomic obstacles.

The problems are chiefly related to identification of the midline. Here it may be pointed out that in scoliotic patients the

Fig. 2.6a. Verification of sagittal direction of spinal needle introduction by observation from two vantage points.

Fig. 2.6b.

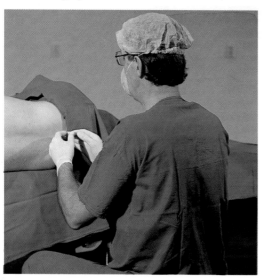

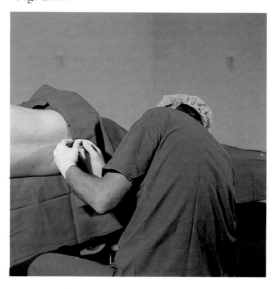

vertebrae are rotated, forcing one to divert somewhat from the perpendicular plane to the back. It is of great help to use two vantage points, 90°(apart, when modifying the direction of the needle and also to use the two-hand "stereotactic" grip (Fig. 2.9).

Not infrequently the bevel of the needle will act as a "rudder" and divert the needle from the midline. In such cases it can be of help to insert the needle through the supra- and interspinous ligaments with the bevel in the transverse plane and rotate the needle 90° just prior to piercing the dura.

When bony contacts are frequently made the direction of the needle must be modified in a systematic way. Provided one is able to keep in the midline, adjustments to a more cephalad or caudad direction are made. For that purpose the needle is withdrawn so that the tip lies subcutaneously, whereupon the new direction is taken up and the puncture attempt repeated.

Fig. 2.7.

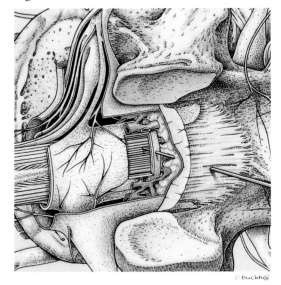

Fig. 2.8. Free flow of CSF.

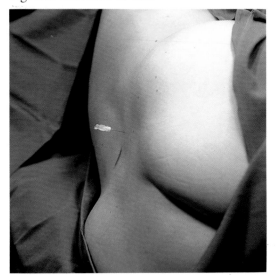

Fig. 2.9. The two-hand, "stereotactic," grip of the spinal needle to facilitate control of minor modifications of needle direction.

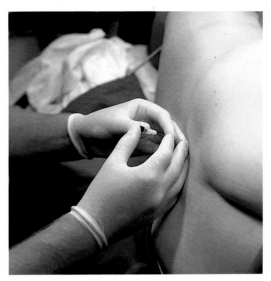

Paramedian approach.

The positioning of the patient is essentially as noted above; however, it is not necessary to flex the back of the patient to the same degree. The paramedian approach might be preferred for patients with a fixed lumbar spine or a scoliosis. Identification of interspaces is made as described above. With the patient in a lateral position the spinal needle is inserted about 2 cm lateral to the midline opposite the dorsal spine of the vertebra caudad to the vertebral interspace to be entered. The needle is advanced in a direction such that its tip will enter the ligamentum flavum near the midline at the next cephalad interspace. This usually requires the needle to be inserted in a cephalad direction at approximately 30° and slightly toward the medial axis of the body. Once the ligamentum flavum is identified the procedure continues as noted for the midline approach above.

Fig. 2.10.

Fig. 2.11. The paramedian approach to the lumbar subarachnoid space.

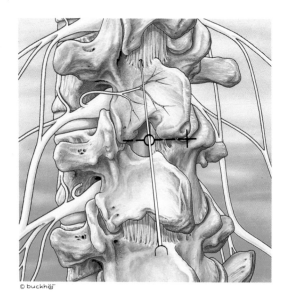

© buckhój

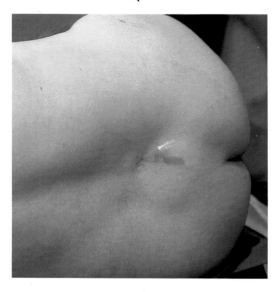

Taylor's approach

Taylor's approach is a modification of the paramedian approach and entails the introduction of the spinal needle through the lumbosacral foramen (L5 – S1 interspace). This technique has definite merits in patients with extremely calcified vertebral ligaments or anatomic aberrations in the lumbar spine.

The needle is introduced through a skin wheal made 1 cm cephalad to and 1 cm medial to the posterior superior iliac spine. It is then advanced in a 45= cephalad and medial direction toward the L5 – S1 interspace in the midline.

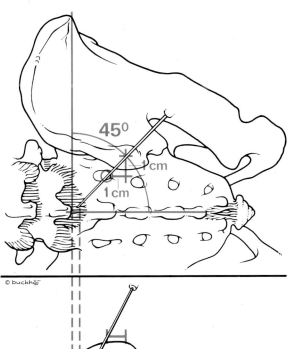

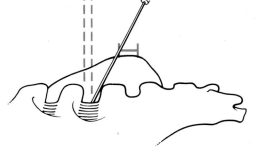

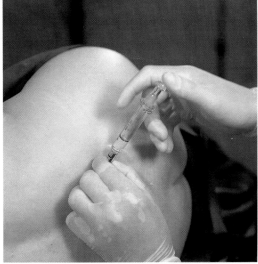

Fig. 2.13. Taylor's approach, spinal needle in position.

Fig. 2.12. Schematic drawing of Taylor's approach to the lumbar subarachnoid space.

99

Continuous technique

The technique of puncture is the same as described above but for this purpose a 17-gauge Tuohy (or similar) needle is used. When piercing the dura/arachnoid the bevel should be longitudinal to the fibers of the dura. After the subarachnoid space is entered the stylet is partially unseated to assure the operator that CSF is flowing freely. The bevel of the needle is pointed cephalad and an epidural catheter advanced 1 – 2 cm into the subarachnoid space. The needle is removed and the catheter secured in place. After the patient is returned to the supine position the chosen spinal anesthetic agent is titrated in to achieve the desired anesthetic level.

The catheter should not be advanced in the face of significant paresthesias. A sterile technique must be maintained at all times during the original procedure as well as for additional injections. Injections should be made through a bacterial filter. With the patient in a fixed supine position the distribution of analgesia could be varied by employing hypobaric or hyperbaric solutions.

This technique was frequently used for vascular procedures in the past but was almost completely replaced by continuous epidural blocks. Recently there has been a rebirth of enthusiasm for the technique. It should also be considered after accidental dural punctures as a result of an unsuccessful attempt to perform an epidural.

Local anesthetic solutions

The local anesthetic solutions that are used for lumbar spinal anesthesia are usually made hyperbaric, i.e., have a higher specific gravity than CSF, by the inclusion of dextrose or glucose. Their specific gravity varies between 1.030 and 1.035. Ordinary plain solutions of local anesthetics are essentially isobaric at room temperature but can be made slightly hypobaric (specific gravity less than 1.007) by warming to 37°C.

A vasopressor can be used as an adjuvant in order to prolong the duration of action, i.e., epinephrine, maximum 0.2 mg. The duration of block in the caudad dermatomes is prolonged by up to 50%.

The duration of analgesia obtained by plain solutions of the different local anesthetics varies a great deal. Lidocaine lasts for 30 – 60 min and mepivacaine for 60 – 90 min whereas tetracaine and bupivacaine work for 120 – 180 min.

The segmental spread of cutaneous analgesia is traditionally considered to be related to the position of the patient during and shortly after the injection and to the amount of local anesthetic injected. Since a hyperbaric local anesthetic solution tends to occupy the most dependent parts of the subarachnoid space the distribution of the block can be determined by the positioning of the patient. However, recent investigations have shown that the positioning of the patient might not be of the predictive importance generally thought. For practical purposes we still recommend consideration of the position of the patient (in reality the position of the spinal canal) when performing the block. For operations involving the leg or inguinal area the spinal is done with the patient in approximately a 10° head-up position; this position is maintained for 2 – 3 min before the patient is returned to supine position, assuming there are no changes in sensorium or vital signs.

The injection of the anesthetic solution should take place only when free flow of CSF through the needle is obtained and after the needle has been rotated 90°. A correct needle position is further verified by free aspiration of CSF before the injection starts as well as after injection of 50% and 100% of the predetermined dose.

The patient is returned to the supine position by gentle lifting so that he does not have to strain or lift his head. The anesthetic level is repeatedly checked by pinprick or alcohol (or similar substance) and the required level obtained by tilting the operating table.

The profundity and duration of block is a function of the amount of drug, the position of the patient, and the speed of injection as well as other factors. For operations involving the leg or inguinal area in an adult patient 10 – 15 mg tetracaine (or 3 ml 0.5% hyperbaric bupivacaine) is ordinarily used, while for elderly individuals the dose should be reduced to around 6 – 10 mg and 2 ml, respectively.

For saddle block analgesia (blockade of the sacral roots only), 3 – 5 mg tetracaine or 1 ml (5 mg) of hyperbaric bupivacaine is injected with the patient in the sitting position, which should be maintained for a minimum of 3 min.

Local anesthetics are almost completely absorbed by the neural tissues within 10 min, after which time the position of the patient can be modified, i.e., to the prone position.

Thoracic spinal block

Midline approach

The patient lies in the lateral position with the head comfortably resting on a small pillow. The thoracic spine is bowed out toward the operator. In the midthoracic area the angulation of the dorsal spines is very acute and the vertebral interspaces often very narrow.

The appropriate dorsal spine is identified by either counting down from the prominent vertebra C7 or up from the lumbar area. A 10-cm 22-gauge spinal needle is inserted through a skin wheal made with a local anesthetic. It is further advanced at an acute angle into the supra- and intraspinous ligaments. The operator should have the feel of the ligamentous structures being penetrated by the needle when it is advanced in the midline. As the deeper layers of the ligaments are encountered, re-sistance to advancing the needle will be slightly increased. Two end-points should be encountered when a 22-gauge needle is used:

1. The entrance of the needle into the epidural space, which will be noted as a slight loss of resistance to advancement

2. The puncture of the dura/arachnoid, which should be done very deliberately

The first end-point should be verified by removing the stylet from the needle and ascertaining that no CSF can be withdrawn. The second end-point, which is usually obvious, should produce a free flow of CSF.

For blocks done below the T9 level, the acuteness of the angle of the needle is modified using a technique which is essentially the same as that described for block in the lumbar area.

Fig. 2.14. Thoracic spinal puncture by the midline approach. Note the angulation of the needle to the skin so as to be parallel to the spinous processes.

Fig. 2.15.

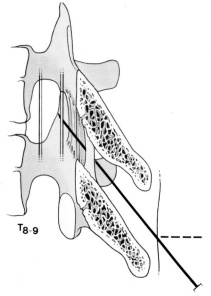

T8-9

© buckhøj

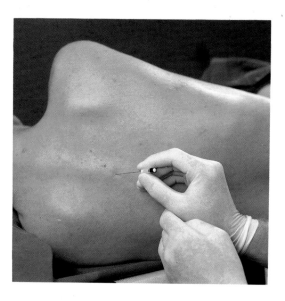

Paramedian approach

Position of the patient and location of the appropriate interspace are the same as noted in the previous section. At a point approximately 1–2 cm lateral to the caudad tip of the dorsal spine which is immediately above the interspace to be entered, a 10-cm 22-gauge spinal needle is inserted perpendicular to the longitudinal axis of the patient and slightly toward the midline. The needle is advanced until the tip hits the vertebral arch. It is then carefully walked off the arch and advanced very slowly until the dura/arachnoid is punctured and CSF appears at the needle hub. The puncturing of the dura/arachnoid is usually an obvious, distinct end-point.

Between 1 and 4 mg of tetracaine, in 1 – 2 ml of either an isobaric or a hyperbaric solution, may be injected. Any comparable local anesthetic solution could be used.

NOTE: Since the spinal cord lies immediately under the dura/arachnoid, piercing of these structures should be done with extreme care. In order to ascertain that the bevel of the needle lies entirely within the subarachnoid space gentle aspiration should produce a free flow of CSF also after rotation of the needle 90°.

Fig. 2.16a. Thoracic spinal puncture by the paramedian approach. The initial direction of the needle is perpendicular to the skin which ensures contact with the vertebral arch.

Fig. 2.16b.

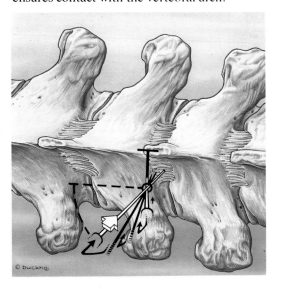

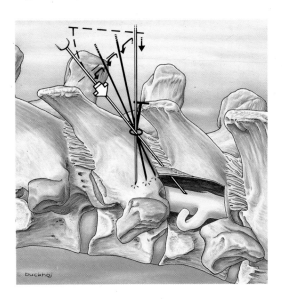

Spinal anesthesia in children

Following induction of light general anesthesia with minimal amounts of ketamine intramuscularly or by low concentrations of inhalational agents, spinal anesthesia is induced at the L4–5 interspace with a 5-cm 25-gauge needle with the patient in the lateral position. After completion of the injection of the local anesthetic, the child is returned to the supine position. Intraoperatively light general anesthesia is maintained with sedative agents, nitrous oxide in oxygen, or minimal doses of ketamine. Endotracheal intubation and/or controlled ventilation is used as necessary. Analgesics or neuromuscular blocking agents are rarely required.

For short-lasting procedures hyperbaric lidocaine solutions may be employed. For patients younger than 3 years 2 mg/kg is given, while for older children decreasing doses down to 1 mg/kg are recommended. For procedures of an estimated duration of up to 90 min, hyperbaric tetracaine is used. For patients below 3 years of age the recommended dose is 1 mg/year of age and for patients older than 3 years 0.2 mg /kg body weight.

Interest in this technique in pediatric patients has renewed recently since it has been reported that various respiratory problems are reduced in comparison with general anesthesia alone.

Postspinal headache

By tradition patients who have undergone a spinal puncture are kept in bed for up to 12 h because of the risk of postspinal headache. We do not concur with this policy, and the literature does not corroborate its validity.

Postspinal headache is distinguished by the fact that it usually appears only when the patient regains an upright position. It is most often localized to the occiput but other presentations are seen. It is usually combined with nausea and dizziness. The cause is considered to be a continuous leakage of CSF through the puncture hole in the dura/arachnoid with concomitant low CSF pressure. This complication is best prevented by using as fine a spinal needle as possible, by puncturing the dura with the bevel of the needle in a longitudinal direction, and by avoiding repeated subarachnoid punctures in attempts to obtain spinal analgesia. The patient should also be kept well hydrated during and after the block.

If a postspinal headache occurs, mild analgesics, hydration, and bed rest are usually sufficient. Should the headache be severe or persist over 3 days, additional measures should be taken. The common denominator of therapy is the prevention of further CSF leakage. The best known technique is to perform an epidural blood patch. This is accomplished by injecting 10 ml of autologous blood, drawn under sterile conditions, into the epidural space at a site close to the original spinal puncture. Very good results have been reported. Some object to this procedure, referring to a risk of local tissue reactions or epidural abscess formation. However, few side effects have been reported although this fact does not exclude a certain complication rate.

An alternative technique is to insert an epidural catheter at the level of the spinal puncture and inject 30 – 50 ml of preservate free saline in the epidural space. Often this alone will relieve the headache. Subsequent injections through the catheter over the next 24 – 48 h might be required. The catheter is removed when the patient has been pain-free and ambulated for 12 h. Most headaches can be cured in this way.

Suggested reading

General

Bengtsson M, Löfström JB, Malmqvist L-Å (1985) Skin conductance responses during spinal analgesia. Acta Anaesthesiol Scand 29:67

Bergmann H (1972) 20 Jahre Spinalanaesthesie. Ein Klinischer Erfahrungsbericht. Der Anaesthesist 21:133

Flaatten H, Raeder J (1985) Spinal anaesthesia for outpatient surgery. Anaesthesia 40:1108

Green NM (1985) Distribution of local anaesthetic solutions within the subarachnoidal space. Anesth Analg 64:715

Löfström JB, Malmqvist L-Å, Bengtsson M (1984) Can the "sympatho-galvanic reflex" (Skin conduction response) be used to evaluate the extent of sympathetic block in spinal analgesia? Acta Anaesthesiol Scand 28:578

Moore DC (1982) Factors influencing spinal anesthesia. Reg Anaesth 7:20

Orko R, Pitkänen M, Rosenberg PH (1986) Subarachnoid anaesthesia with 0.75% bupivacaine in patients with chronic renal failure. Br J Anaesth 58:605

Mukkada TA, Bridenbaugh PO, Singh P et al (1986) Effects of dose, volume and concentration of glucose-free bupivacaine in spinal anesthesia. Reg Anesth 11:98

Rocco AG, Raymond SA, Murray E et al. (1985) Differential spread of blockade to touch, cold, and pinprick during spinal anesthesia. Anesth Analg 64:917

Smith TC (1968) The lumbar spine and subarachnoid block. Anesthesiology 29:60

Stratmann D, Götte A, Meyer-Hamme K et al (1979) Klinische Verläufe von über 6000 Spinalanästhesien mit Bupivacain. Reg Anaesth 2:49

Wildsmith JAW, Rocco AG (1985) Current concepts in spinal anesthesia. Reg Anaesth 10:119

Drugs

Bengtsson M, Edström HH, Löfström JB (1983) Spinal analgesia with bupivacaine, mepivacaine and tetracaine. Acta Anaesthesiol Scand 27:278

Bigler D, Hjortsö NC, Edström H et al (1986) Comparative effects of intrathecal bupivacaine and tetracaine on analgesia, cardiovascular function and plasma catecholamines. Acta Anaesthesiol Scand 30:199

Burm AG, van Kleef JW, Gladines MP et al (1983) Plasma concentrations of lidocaine and bupivacaine after subarachnoid administration. Anesthesiology 59:191

Chambers WA, Littlewood DG, Logan MR et al (1981) Effect of added epinephrine on spinal anesthesia with lidocaine. Anesth Analg 60:417

Chambers WA, Littlewood DG, Scott DB (1982) Spinal anaesthesia with hyperbaric bupivacaine: effect of added vasoconstrictors. Anesth Analg 61:49

Chambers WA, Littlewood DG, Edström HH et al (1982) Spinal anaesthesia with hyperbaric bupivacaine. Br J Anaesthesiol 54:75

Cozian A, Pinaud M, Lepage JY et al (1986) Effects of meperidine spinal anesthesia on hemodynamics, plasma catecholamines, angiotensin I, aldosterone and histamine concentrations in elderly men. Anesthesiology 66:815

Famewo CE, Naguib M (1985) Spinal anaesthesia with meperidine as the sole agent. Can Anaesth Soc J 32:533

Green NM (1983) Uptake and elimination of local anesthetics during spinal anesthesia. Anesth Analg 62:1013

Leicht CH, Carlsson SA (1986) Prolongation of lidocaine spinal anesthesia with epinephrine and phenylephrine. Anesth Analg 65:365

Rocco AG, Concepcion M, Sheskey M et al. (1984) A double-blind evaluation of intrathecal bupivacaine without glucose and a standard solution of hyperbaric tetracaine. Reg Anesth 9:1

Sheskey MC, Rocco AG, Bizzari-Schmid M et al (1983) A dose-response study of bupivacaine for spinal anesthesia. Anesth Analg 62:931

Tattersall MP (1983) Isobaric bupivacaine and hyperbaric amethocaine for spinal analgesia. Anaesthesia 38:115

van Kleef JW, Burm AGL (1984) Effects of adrenaline during epidural and spinal anaesthesia. In: van Kleef JW, Burm AGL, Spierdijk J (eds) Current concepts in regional anaesthesia. Proceedings of the second general meeting of the European Society of Regional Anaesthesia. Martinus Nijhoff, The Hague, p 174

Distribution of block

Axelsson K, Widman B (1979) Clinical significance of specific gravity of spinal anaesthetic agents. Acta Anaesthesiol Scand 23:427

Axelsson KH, Edström HH, Sundberg AEA et al (1982) Spinal anaesthesia with hyperbaric 0.5% bupivacaine: effects of volume. Acta Anaesthesiol Scand 26:439

Axelsson KH, Edström HH, Widman GB (1984) Spinal anaesthesia with glucose-free 0.5% bupivacaine: effects of different volumes. Br J Anaesthesiol 56:271

Cameron AE, Arnold RW, Ghorisa MW et al (1981) Spinal analgesia using bupivacaine 0.5% plain. Variations in the extent of block with patient age. Anesthesia 36:318

Chambers WA, Edström HH, Scott D (1981) Effect of baricity on spinal anaesthesia with bupivacaine. Br J Anaesthesiol 53:279

Kalso E, Tuominen M, Rosenberg PH (1982) Effect of posture and some CSF characteristics on spinal anaesthesia with isobaric 0.5% bupivacaine. Br J Anaesthesiol 54:1179

Kennedy WF (1978) Effects of baricity, position, and equipment on successful spinal anesthesia. Reg Anesth 3:2

Levin E, Muravchick S, Gold MI (1981) Isobaric tetracaine spinal anesthesia and the lithotomy position. Anesth Analg 60:810

McClure JH, Brown DT, Wildsmith JAW (1982) Effect of injected volume and speed of injection on the spread of spinal anaesthesia with isobaric amethocaine. Br J Anaesth 54:917

McCulloch WJD, Littlewood DG (1986) Influence of obesity on spinal analgesia with isobaric 0.5% bupivacaine. Br J Anaesth 58:610

Mukkada T, Bridenbaugh PO, Sing P (1983) Clinical effects of dose vs volume in isobaric bupivacaine spinal anesthesia. Reg Anaesth 8:50

Park WY, Balingit PE, MacNamara E (1975) Effects of patient age, pH of cerebrospinal fluid and vasopressors on onset and duration of spinal anesthesia. Anesth Analg 43:455

Pitkänen M, Hapaniemi L, Tuominen M et al (1984) Influence of age on spinal anesthesia with isobaric 0.5% bupivacaine. Br J Anaesthesiol 56:279

Pitkänen M, Tuominen M, Asantila R et al (1985) Effect of aspiration of cerebro-spinal fluid on spinal anaesthesia with isobaric 0.5% bupivacaine. Acta Anaesthesiol Scand 29:590

Sinclair CJ, Scott DB, Edström HH (1982) Effect of the Trendelenburg position on spinal anaesthesia with hyperbaric bupivacaine. Br J Anaesth 54:497

Sundnes KO, Vaagenes P, Skretting P et al (1982) Spinal analgesia with hyperbaric bupivacaine: effects of volume of solution. Br J Anaesth 54:69

Tuominen M, Kalso E, Rosenberg PH (1982) Effects of posture on the spread of spinal anaesthesia with isobaric 0.75% or 0.5% bupivacaine. Br J Anaesth 54:313

Spinal anesthesia in infants

Abajian C, Mellish RWP, Brown AF et al (1984) Spinal anesthesia for surgery in the high risk infant. Anesth Analg 63:359

Berkowitz S, Greene BA (1984) Spinal anesthesia in children: report based on 350 patients under 13 years of age. Anesthesiology 12:376

Blaise G, Roy WL (1984) Spinal anesthesia in children. Anesth Analg 63:1840

Gleason CA, Martin RJ, Anderson JW et al (1983) Optimal position for a spinal tap in preterm infants. Pediatrics 71:31

Harnik EV, Hoy GR, Potolicchio S et al (1986) Spinal anesthesia in premature infants recovering from respiratory distress syndrome. Anesthesiology 64:95

Majhew JF, Moreno L (1984) Spinal anesthesia for the high risk neonate. Anesth Analg 63:782

Schulte-Steinberg O (1984) Regional anaesthesia for children. Ann Chir Gynec 73:158

Slater HM, Stephen CR (1950) Hypobaric pontocaine spinal anaesthesia in children. Anesthesiology 11:709

Spencer HT, Barnes PJ (1980) Spinal anaesthesia for pediatric radiotherapy. Anaesth Intensive Care 8:214

Complications

General

Bert AA, Laasberg LH (1985) Aseptic meningitis following spinal anesthesia – a complication of the past? Anesthesiology 62:674.

Blacker HM (1971) The dangers of lumbar puncture in the presence of an intracranial mass lesion. Clin Med 78:21

Brem SS, Hafler DA, van Uitert RL et al (1981) Spinal subarachnoid hematoma. A hazard of lumbar puncture resulting in reversible paraplegia. N Engl J Med. 305:1020

Eerola M, Kaukinen L, Kaukinen S (1981) Fatal brain lesion following spinal anaesthesia. Report of a case. Acta Anaesthesiol Scand 25:115

Jonsson LO, Einarsson P, Olsson GL (1983) Subdural haematoma and spinal anaesthesia. Anaesthesia 38:144

Kane BE (1981) Neurological deficits following epidural or spinal anesthesia. Anesth Analg 60:150

Kleinman B, Belusko R (1986) Delayed cephalad spread of a lidocaine spinal anesthetic causing ventilatory failure. Anesth Analg 65:523

Kortum K, Rössler B, Nolte H (1979) Morbidität nach Spinalanaesthesie. Reg Anaesth 2:5

Koster H, Weintrob M (1930) Complications of spinal anesthesia. Am J Surg VIII(6):1165

Mattingly SB, Stanton-Hicks M (1981) Low-dose heparin therapy and spinal anesthesia. Question and Answers. JAMA 246:886

Messer HD, Forshan VR, Brust JCM et al (1976) Transient paraplegia from hematoma after lumbar puncture. A consequence of anticoagulant therapy. JAMA 235:529

Newrick P, Read D (1982) Subdural haematoma as a complication of spinal anaesthetic. Br Med J 285:341

Noble AB, Murray JG (1971) A review of the complications of spinal anesthesia with experiences in Canadian teaching hospitals from 1959 to 1969. Can Anaesth Soc J 18:5

Panning B, Mehler D, Lehnhardt E (1983) Transient low-frequency hypoacousia after spinal anaesthesia. Lancet 2:582

Pearce JMS (1982) Hazards of lumbar puncture. Brit Med J 285:1521

Phillips OC, Ebner H, Nelson T et al (1969) Neurologic complications following spinal anaesthesia with lidocaine: a prospective review of 10,440 cases. Anesthesiology 30:284

Plötz J, Schreiber W (1984) Intrazerebrale Massenblutung und Arteria-spinalis-anterior-Syndrom in ursächlichem Zusammenhang mit rückenmarksnahen Betäubungsverfahren? – Zwei Fallbeschreibungen. Anästh Intensivther Notfallmed 19:307

Rudehill A, Gordon E, Rahn T (1983) Subdural haematoma. A rare but life-threatening complication after spinal anaesthesia. Acta Anaesthesiol Scand 27:376

Sadjadpour K (1977) Hazards of anticoagulation therapy shortly after lumbar puncture. JAMA 237:1692

Schou J, Scherb M (1986) Postoperative sagittal sinus thrombosis after spinal anesthesia. Anesth Analg 65:539

Sinclair DM (1973) Failure of 4 successive spinal anaesthetics. S Afr Med J 47:1984

van Deripe DR, Yim GKW (1960) Local anesthetic activity of partially hydrolyzed solutions of tetracaine hydrochloride. Anesthesiology 21:26

Wolf S, Spielman F, Teeple E (1981) Spinal subarachnoid hematoma after lumbar puncture. N Engl J Med 305:699

Postspinal headache

Bridenbaugh PO (1978) Postdural puncture headache. Reg Anesth 5:8

Jarvis AP, Greenawalt JW, Fagraeus L (1986) Intravenous caffeine for postdural puncture headache. Anesth Analg 65:316

Jones RJ (1974) The role of recumbency in the prevention and treatment of postspinal headache. Anesth Analg 53:788

Mihic DN (1985) Postspinal headache and relation of needle bevel to longitudinal dural fibers. Reg Anesth 10:76

Poukkula E (1984) The problem of post-spinal headache. Ann Chir Gynaecol 73:139

Usubiaga JE, Usibiaga LE, Brea LM et al (1967) Effect of saline injections on epidural and subarachnoid space pressures and relation to postspinal anesthesia headache. Anesth Analg 46:293

Vandam LD, Dripps RD (1956) Long-term follow-up of patients who received 10098 spinal anesthetics: syndrome of decreased intracranial pressure. JAMA 161:81

Epidural blood patch

Abouleish E, de la Vega S, Blendinger I et al (1975) Long-term follow-up of epidural blood patch. Anesth Analg 54:459

Cohen SE (1985) Epidural blood patch in outpatients: a simpler approach. Anesth Analg 64:458

Crawford SJ (1985) Epidural blood patch. Anaesthesia 40:381

Loeser EA, Bennett GM, Sederberg JH et al (1978) Time versus success rate for epidural blood patch. Anesthesiology 49:147

Rainbird A, Pfitzner J (1983) Restricted spread of analgesia following epidural blood patch. Case report with a review of possible complications. Anaesthesia 38:481

Rao TLK (1985) Temporary relief of postlumbar puncture headache with epidural blood patch. Reg Anasth 10:191

Ravindran RS (1984) Epidural autologous blood patch on an outpatient basis. Anesth Analg 63:962

Rosenberg PH, Heavner JE (1985) In vitro study of the effect of epidural blood patch on leakage through a dural puncture. Anesth Analg 64:501

Szeinfeld M, Ihmeidan I, Moser MM et al (1986) Epidural blood patch: evaluation of the volume and spread of the blood injected into the epidural space. Anaesthesiology 64:820

Lumbar epidural block

Puncture of the lumbar epidural space can be accomplished by either a midline or a paramedian approach.

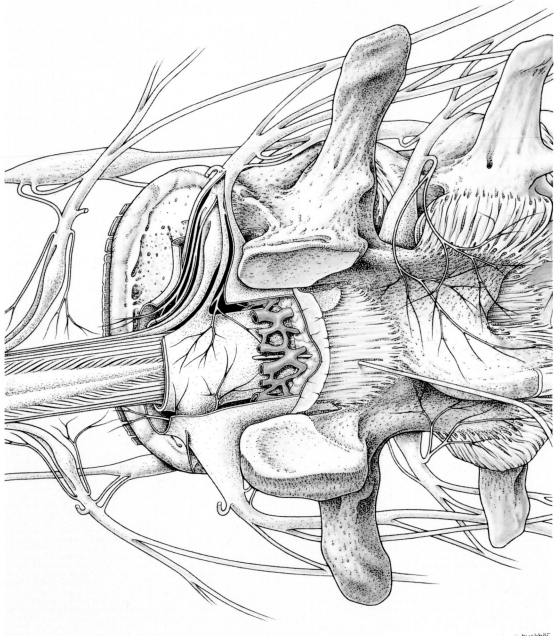

Fig. 2.17.

Midline approach

The positioning of the patient and the initial steps of the procedure are essentially the same as described for lumbar spinal anesthesia. However, a Tuohy needle is used instead of a spinal needle. When the deeper portions of the interspinous ligament are entered, the stylet is removed and a 5-ml syringe with low resistance, filled with normal saline or air, is attached. It is important to avoid any contamination of the plunger with talcum powder from the operator's gloves as this will increase the friction within the syringe rendering evaluation of loss of resistance difficult or impossible.

The left hand grips the Luer-Loc fitting of the syringe filled with normal saline between the first and second digits and support is gained by resting the knuckles against the back of the patient (Bromage's grip, Fig 2.19). The right hand is prepared to press the plunger. With both hands working together – the controlling role of the left being the most important – the needle is continuously advanced with extreme care at the same time as the right hand firmly presses the plunger. A sudden, very obvious, loss of resistance to injection indicates that the epidural space has been entered. The advancement of the needle should be stopped at this stage to avoid dural puncture.

When employing a syringe filled with air, the initial steps of the procedure are as described above. However, the needle is carefully advanced in a stepwise fashion, and after each advancement the resistance to injection of air is evaluated by ballottement of the plunger. When there is a sudden loss of resistance the epidural space has been entered.

Fig. 2.18. Lumbar epidural puncture by the midline approach. The direction of the needle is identical with that in lumbar spinal block.

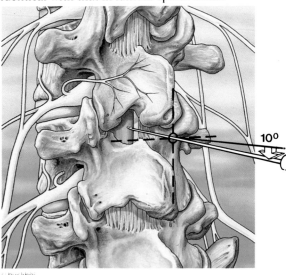

Fig. 2.19. Bromage's grip.

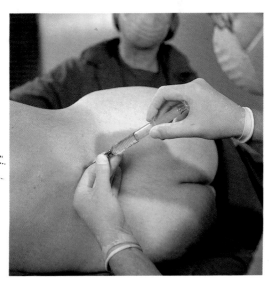

Paramedian approach

With the patient in a lateral position a skin wheal is raised 1 – 2 cm lateral to the cephalad border of the dorsal spine of the vertebra just caudad to the vertebral interspace to be entered. Generous infiltration anesthesia of the skin and soft tissue is obtained by means of a 70-mm 22-gauge needle directed 10–15° to the longitudinal axis of the patient and toward the midline. Bony contact with the vertebral arch of the cephalad vertebra is accomplished. At this point a further few milliliters of the local anesthetic are injected and the smaller needle removed. A Tuohy needle is then inserted through a small nick in the skin and advanced as above until bony contact is obtained. The needle is then walked off the vertebral arch in a cephalad direction to a point when the bone is replaced by an elastic ligamentous contact. The stylet is removed and a syringe filled with air or normal saline is attached. The needle is carefully introduced into the ligamentum flavum. When loss of resistance (see above) is obtained the local anesthetic is injected or an epidural catheter is inserted.

Continuous technique

Any of the above-described techniques can be used with the following changes. A thin-walled 17-gauge Tuohy or similar needle is used. With identification of the epidural space the bevel of the needle is directed cephalad. A catheter is then advanced 2 – 3 cm beyond the tip of the needle. The needle is removed and the catheter secured in place.

Some clinicians prefer to inject the initial dose of the local anesthetic before threading the epidural catheter in order to expand the epidural space and thereby avoid intravascular positioning of the catheter (Fig. 4.12b).

Fig. 2.20. Lumbar epidural puncture by the paramedian approach. Point of skin puncture and modifications of direction of the needle as it walks off the vertebral arch of the nearest cephalad vertebra.

Fig. 2.21. The width of the epidural space can be increased by the injection of a local anesthetic prior to the introduction of the epidural catheter.

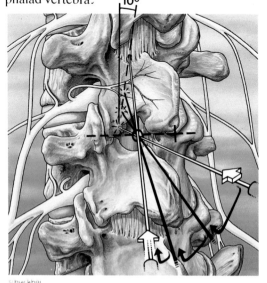

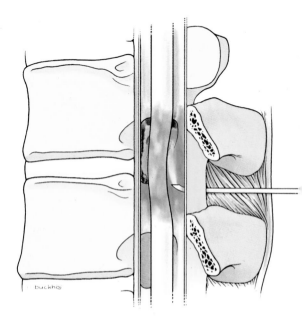

Thoracic epidural block

The following anatomic differences in relation to the lumbar area must be kept in mind:

1. The dorsal spine of a thoracic vertebra is angulated in relation to the vertebral body (p 10).

2. The spinal medulla usually ends at the L1 or L2 level, so for punctures above this level there is always a risk of mechanical damage to the cord.

3. The thickness of the ligamentum flavum and the epidural space is considerably less, which makes loss of resistance less evident and increases the risk of dural puncture.

From this it follows that thoracic epidural anesthesia is technically more demanding than lumbar epidural anesthesia and that the procedure is associated with certain risks of mechanical damage to the medulla.

While gaining experience in thoracic epidurals one should select the technique with the highest success rate and the fewest complications. According to our experience the paramedian technique, employing loss of resistance with normal saline or air, best fulfills these criteria.

Fig. 2.22. A midthoracic vertebra. Note angulation of the spinous process.

Fig. 2.23. Angulation of needle for thoracic epidural puncture by the midline approach.

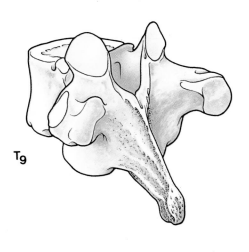

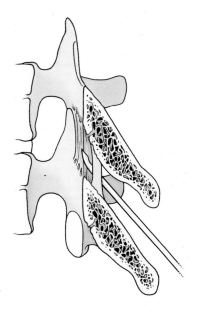

Paramedian approach

The dorsal spines of the appropriate inter-space are identified by counting down from C7. One to two centimeters lateral to the caudad border of the cephalad dorsal spine a skin wheal is raised with local anesthetic. Through this wheal a 70-mm 22-gauge needle is inserted perpendicular to the skin during infiltration analgesia with 5 ml or less of a dilute local anesthetic solution. Bony contact with the vertebral arch of the caudad vertebra of the interspace is sought. The needle is then gently redirected cephalad and slightly medially under continuous infiltration anesthesia until bone contact is lost. The tip of the needle is then just above the ligamentum flavum. The depth and direction is noted and the needle removed. A small nick, 2 – 3 mm long, is then made in the skin wheal and a Touhy needle (16 – 18 gauge) carefully inserted in a perpendicular direction toward the vertebral arch. With the direction of the prior needle in mind, the Tuohy needle is gently walked off the lamina in a cephalad

direction until bone contact is lost. Frequently a distinct ligamentous contact is not noticed. At this stage the stylet is removed and a glass syringe filled with normal saline or air is attached. The left hand grips the Luer-Loc fitting with Bromage's grip.

The right hand is prepared to press the plunger. With both hands working together – the controlling role of the left being the most important – the needle is advanced with extreme care at the same time as the right hand firmly presses the plunger. At this initial stage there is usually only a slight resistance since the ligamentum flavum has not been entered. Not infrequently resistance to injection is not obtained until the needle is advanced somewhat.

In a typical case resistance to injection should ensue after advancing the needle 3 – 5 mm (occasionally up to 1 cm). After further advancement (3 – 10 mm) a sudden loss of resistance occurs, indicating that the epidural space has been entered. The maneuver must be extremely well controlled and the role of the left hand must be stressed.

Fig. 2.24a. Thoracic epidural puncture by the paramedian approach. The needle is initially directed perpendicular to the skin to ensure primary contact with the vertebral arch.

Fig. 2.24b

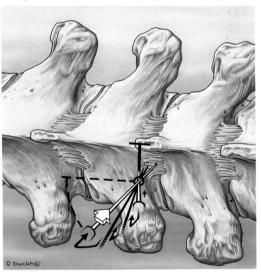

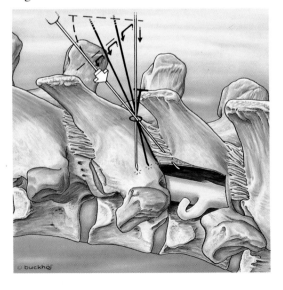

In many cases renewed bone contact is obtained; the needle is then redirected more cephalad or caudad. Especially in the T5 – T8 region the interspaces between the vertebral arches are so narrow that epidural puncture in some instances cannot be obtained. Attempts should therefore primarily be made above or below this region.

Not infrequently there is no obvious change in resistance to injection as the needle is advanced. This is probably due to the fact that the ligamentum flavum is so thin that the entirety of the bevel of the needle is never within the ligament at the same time. It is therefore recommended that if there is any suspicion whatsoever that the epidural space has been entered, one should attempt to advance an epidural catheter. In the experience of the authors, if the catheter can be introduced 3 cm without significant resistance then it lies within the epidural space. If the catheter cannot be inserted, the catheter and the needle are removed together and a new attempt made. The catheter should never be removed through the needle as the catheter can be cut off.

Fig. 2.25. Thoracic epidural puncture by the midline approach. Point of skin puncture in relation to spinous processes and angulation of needle in relation to the perpendicular plane.

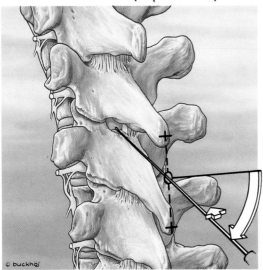

Midline approach

The patient is positioned and the appropriate vertebral interspace identified as for thoracic spinal block. An 18-gauge, thin-walled Tuohy or similar needle is inserted in the midline at a very acute angle, anywhere from 35 – 60°. The loss of resistance technique is used to identify the epidural space. The interspinous ligaments and the ligamentum flavum can be identified by ballottement of the plunger of an air-filled glass syringe or by constant pressure at the plunger of a syringe filled with normal saline as the needle is advanced through the interspace. There is usually a sudden loss of resistance when the epidural space is entered. In other cases the ligamentum flavum is poorly defined as described (under "Paramedian approach") above.

The above-described techniques apply to punctures above the T9 level. For punctures below that level the technique is simpler and in essence the same as described for lumbar epidural block. Below T9, the ligamentum flavum is generally distinct so that a more evident loss of resistance is obtained in most cases.

Even in experienced hands puncture of the thoracic epidural space may occasionally be difficult. Considering the risk of damage to the cord, the procedure should not be tried until one has considerable experience with lumbar epidural blocks and preferably under the guidance of a colleague experienced in thoracic epidural analgesia. Indications for thoracic epidural blockade are rarely absolute. If problems are encountered during attempts to perform the block it is recommended that one seek the assistance of a more experienced colleague at an early stage or that one gives up the attempts and considers other therapeutic approaches.

Comparison of the paramedian and the midline approach

In comparison with the midline technique the paramedian approach to the epidural space has the following distinct advantages:

1. The first rigid structure met by the needle is the vertebral arch and not the deep supra- and interspinous ligaments. In this way the position of the tip of the needle in relation to the ligamentum flavum is more adequately controlled.

2. The interspinous ligaments might contain cavities as a result of degenerative changes, which can give a false sensation of loss of resistance.

3. The paramedian approach is more useful in patients who cannot be adequately flexed for any reason.

In the lumbar area the following additional advantages apply:

4. By entering the ligamentum flavum in an oblique direction one will usually experience a more evident loss of resistance as the total length of the bevel of the needle will be contained within the ligament (Figs 2.26 and 2.27).

5. The distance that the needle can be introduced from the position in which loss of resistance was obtained to a depth at which there is a risk of dural puncture will be almost 50% longer when the paramedian approach is used (Fig 2.28).

6. With the more oblique direction of the needle in the paramedian technique the epidural catheter is inserted parallel to the epidural space (Fig 2.28). It has been suggested that this will decrease the incidence of unwanted location of the catheter (i.e., along the anterior aspect of the dural sac).

Fig. 2.26.

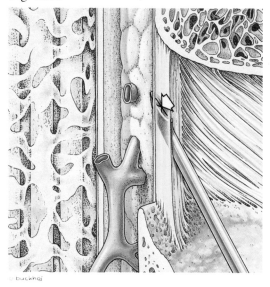

Fig. 2.27.

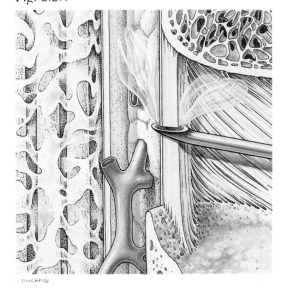

7. With the oblique approach to the epidural space the blunt curvature and not the sharp point of the tip of the Tuohy needle will be the part of the needle most likely to come into contact with the ligamentum flavum (Fig 2.28). Thereby the risk of dural puncture is further minimized.

Verification of epidural puncture

If the epidural catheter can be introduced through the needle without any significant resistance it should be located in the epidural space. However, unrecognized advancement into the subarachnoid space is a possibility. In order to avoid a total spinal block subarachnoid positioning must be excluded.

Obviously, if clear fluid pours out of the needle or begins to rise in the epidural catheter, subarachnoid placement must be suspected. This can be proven by noting the temperature of the fluid (CSF would be at body temperature) and testing the fluid for glucose content. These steps become necessary only if there is any confusion as to the origin of the fluid, i.e., when a saline-filled syringe is used for performing the loss of resistance maneuver. When a subarachnoid puncture has occurred, and one does not want to employ either a single shot or continuous spinal anesthetic, a new attempt at epidural puncture could be made at one interspace cephalad.

Proper positioning of the catheter can also be verified by noting the response to the administration of a test dose of 3 – 5 ml of a local anesthetic containing adrenaline. After administration in the thoracic epidural space this amount causes sensory loss of at least several dermatomes within 2 – 3 min. In contrast, in the lumbar epidural space, minimal if any analgesia will be produced. However, this test dose will cause sensory loss if the catheter is subarachnoid and the presence of adrenaline will produce tachycardia if the catheter has been threaded intravascularly by mistake.

Fig. 2.28.

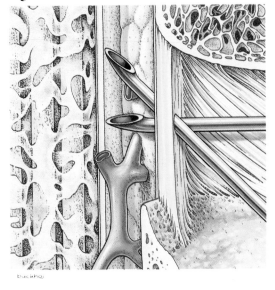

Fig. 2.29.

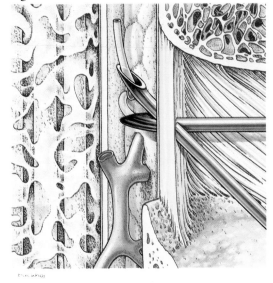

If blood does appear in the catheter, one must consider the possibility of intravascular placement. Any local anesthetic then injected might cause systemic toxicity. To withdraw the catheter from a suspected intravascular position one way to proceed is as follows:

The catheter is attached to a syringe filled with normal saline and pulled back about 1 cm; 1–2 ml of normal saline are injected. The catheter is then aspirated very gently. If there is no backflow of blood the syringe is detached and the hub of the catheter is lowered to below the level of the spinal canal in the dependent position. Occasionally this method produces blood from an intravascular placement that aspiration was unable to determine. Assuming that the above procedures were negative, injection of the test dose of an adrenaline-containing anesthetic is performed while constantly observing the heart rate. If the injection results in an increase in heart rate the position of the catheter is intravascular. If no increase in heart rate is observed the position is most likely extravascular.

Sometimes paresthesias are elicited by introduction of the catheter or the injection of the local anesthetic. In these cases the catheter must be considered to be in an unsuitable position – i.e., in a root sleeve – and the positioning must be adjusted. Do not inject a full dose when paresthesias are obtained.

Never pull the catheter back through the needle as this involves considerable risk of shearing the catheter off.

Choice of local anesthetic agent

Various concentrations of various local anesthetics result in differing degrees and durations of block as well as different risks of systemic toxicity. It is therefore important to select the local anesthetic solution for a specific purpose.

For intraoperative anesthesia we use 2% solutions of mepivacaine or lidocaine with adrenaline, 5 μg/ml, when significant muscle relaxation is needed. Prilocaine is significantly less toxic but not suitable for continuous techniques because of the possibility of methemoglobinemia. Etidocaine 1.5% with adrenaline, 5 μg/ml, has a very rapid onset and produces profound muscle relaxation. We use it occasionally as an "induction agent" but rarely in continuous blocks as very prolonged motor blocks may occur. Bupivacaine 0.5% with adrenaline is another choice that results in an excellent sensory block but in a rather poor motor block. Mixtures of various local anesthetics are controversial and should rarely be used.

For postoperative analgesia we use almost exclusively bupivacaine 0.25% – 0.5%, plain or with adrenaline, which results in minimal motor block.

Calculation of dose

For calculation of the appropriate dose of the chosen local anesthetic one should consider the number of dermatomes that must be blocked in order to obtain adequate analgesia, their localization in relation to the puncture level and patient-related factors such as age and concomitant disease.

The number of dermatomes that have to be blocked in order to make the operation pain-free can be calculated from data given in Chap. 1. As an aid the following suggestions can be made:

Table 2. Segmental distribution of block.

Procedure	Segmental distribution of block
Proctologic procedures	S1 – S5
Operations on the urethra and external genitals	S1 – S5
Operations on the bladder and lower ureters	T8 – S4
Operations on the lower extremities	T10 – S3
Inguinal herniorraphies	T8 – L3
Lower laparotomies	T6 – L2
Upper laparotomies	T4 – T12
Thoracotomies	T1 – T10

The injected local anesthetic spreads in a cephalad and caudad direction from the site of injection. In the thoracic region the spread is essentially symmetrical, in the lumbar area it is chiefly cephalad, and in the caudal area entirely cephalad.

If the epidural block for a lower laparotomy is made at the L3 – L4 level the local anesthetic has to spread ten vertebral levels or segments in the cephalad direction to reach T6, in order to exert the intended effects. In order to do so it will, however, also spread in a caudad direction. For practical purposes one can calculate that the spread takes place in a symmetrical manner. The remaining caudad segments (L4 – S5) thus have to be included in the block in order to obtain a cephalad spread to the T6 level. This means that a total of 17 segments must be included in the block.

If on the other hand the epidural puncture is performed at the T10 – T11 level five segments cephalad to the puncture and five segments caudad to it, i.e., a total of just ten segments, must be included in the block in order to obtain the desired distribution.

The dose of the local anesthetic needed to block the innervation of one dermatome, the segmental dose, is 1.5 – 2.0 ml of the mentioned solutions for a 20- to 40-year-old individual of 175 cm height. The size of the segmental dose is, however, influenced by a number of factors, of which the following are the most important:

1. **Age of the patient**
   a) Children require a segmental dose of 0.1 ml/year.
   b) The segmental dose for individuals over 40 years of age should be reduced by 0.01 ml/year.

2. **Height of the patient**
   For any body height above or below 175 cm the segmental dose should be increased or reduced, respectively, by 0.1 ml/5 cm.

For example, the dose reduction for a patient 84 years old and 152 cm tall is calculated as follows: (84 minus 40) times 0.01 + (175 minus 152) times 0.1/5. The segmental dose should thus be reduced by 0.9 ml.

3. **Pregnancy**
   It is generally recommended that the segmental dose for patients in the third trimester is reduced by 30%.

4. **Advanced arteriosclerosis**
   It is recommended that the calculated segmental dose be reduced by as much as 40% – 50%

5. **Site of injection**
   The suggested segmental dose must be reduced when the dose is administered in the thoracic epidural space in order to avoid a too wide distribution of the resulting block and thereby the risks of arterial hypotension. For low thoracic epidurals the dose should be reduced by 30% – 50% and for high thoracic epidurals by 50% – 75%.

6. Patient-related factors

In the calculation of the total dose some additional, patient-related factors of importance for toxicity of the local anesthetic should be included:

a) Acidosis increases the risk of toxicity as the cellular uptake of the local anesthetic is increased.

b) Cardiac decompensation is associated with reduced hepatic metabolism of the local anesthetic and higher plasma concentrations following epidural administration.

7. Adrenaline

Inclusion of adrenaline, 5 μg/ml, in the local anesthetic solution will decrease systemic absorption and thereby reduce the risk of toxicity. In addition adrenaline increases the spread, intensity, and duration of block and perhaps protects against cardiac toxicity. This adjuvant has at least two drawbacks, however. The pH of premixed, commercial solutions is low, which affects the ionization of the local anesthetic with repeated administration, and the concomitant arterial hypotension is more profound than when plain solutions are used.

From the above follows that the calculation of the appropriate segmental dose in an individual case is associated with certain sources of error. We therefore recommend that the segmental dose is titrated for each patient. This is accomplished by using an epidural catheter and initially a segmental dose of approximately 75% of the calculated value. The resulting block is evaluated after 10 min and supplemented, if necessary, with an additional dose. For simplicity, the size of the supplementary dose can be calculated from the effects of the initial dose: the segmental dose in a particular patient is calculated from the size of the initial dose and the distribution of the resulting anesthesia. The additional number of segments that should be blocked is estimated.

The size of the supplementary dose is the product of these two values. This is a very crude way of determining the total dose requirement in an individual patient. Its application on a routine basis will, however, prevent a significant number of cases complicated by arterial hypotension.

In the very elderly or arteriosclerotic patient we recommend that the calculated dose be administered in two steps, half of it initially followed by the second half 10–15 min later. Thereby two common problems with epidural anesthesia in this group of patients are reduced, namely a too wide distribution and a poor intensity of the block.

Prolongation of epidural analgesia

An epidural block can be prolonged either by continuous administration or by intermittent top-up dosages of a local anesthetic through a catheter. It is our experience that prolongation by intermittent administration results in maintenance of a more profound block than continuous administration. On the other hand, intermittent administration might require more work and is more often associated with cardiovascular instability.

Top-up doses should always be administered before the initial block has regressed significantly. In this way the influence of tachyphylaxis – which will always occur – will be delayed. For intraoperative use of short-acting local anesthetics a dosage interval of 60 min is recommended, while for the long-acting agents the interval should not exceed 120 min. However, for etidocaine this interval may sometimes be too long.

The size of the top-up dose should be adjusted to the age and size of the patient and to the injection level. For a lumbar epidural as little as 3 ml may be required for a small, elderly patient and up to 10 ml for a tall athlete. For a high thoracic epidural the dose is significantly decreased – it should never exceed 4 ml as otherwise arterial hypotension invariably results at some stage. When prolongation by continuous administration of a local anesthetic is employed the hourly maintenance dose will be the same as described for top-up doses.

Tachyphylaxis occurs regularly in thoracic epidurals. In order to reduce its clinical significance it is important to evaluate the distribution of cutaneous analgesia resulting from each subsequent dose and to modify the size of the top-up dose and/or the dosage interval.

Evaluation of epidural analgesia

The distribution of the sensory block is evaluated by pinprick, alcohol, or ethyl chloride. Preferably a blunt needle should be used to avoid puncture wounds. Each dermatome on both sides is tested every 5 min initially, and later every 15th minute. For practical purposes it is sufficient to test only the first 10–15 min after injection. For scientific or teaching purposes an "epiduralogram" might be constructed on which the time for disappearance and reappearance of pinprick or sensation of cold in each dermatome can be stated. From such an "epiduralogram" the following information can be obtained:

- Latency to initial onset (four dermatomes)
- Latency to maximal distribution of cutaneous analgesia
- Latency to regression by two segments from maximal distribution
- Latency to complete regression
- Number of segments blocked by the administered dose
- Amount of local anesthetic per blocked segment
- Number of "segment-minutes" for the administered amount of local anesthetic

The sympathetic block is evaluated by various measurements of the cutaneous temperature, plethysmographs, the somatogalvanic response, the ninhydrin test, or combined laser–doppler methods. Generally the distribution of the sympathetic block on the thorax or abdomen is very difficult to evaluate. From a practical point of view these measurements are restricted to the extremities.

Table 3. The intensity of the motor block is most frequently classified according to Bromage.

No block	Degree IV	Intact flexion of knee and ankle joints
Partial block	Degree III	Subject able to raise knees but not feet from the bed
Almost complete block	Degree II	Subject able to move feet but unable to raise knees
Complete block	Degree I	Subject unable to move legs or feet

Lumbar epidural block in small children

The technique is essentially the same as has been described for adults. However, the puncture should be performed with the child under light general anesthesia and a thinner (19 gauge) Touhy needle should be used. For continuous blocks a 24 gauge polyurethane catheter can be used.

For low laparotomies, urogenital procedures and orthopedic operations on the lower limb the mean dose requirement is 0.5 – 0.7 ml/kg of 0.25% bupivacaine, with or without adrenaline.

Epidural anesthesia is used intraoperatively in order to allow for a more superficial level of general anesthesia and postoperatively for pain relief. For maintenance of the block a continuous injection, by means of a precision pump, of 0.08 ml/kg/0.25% bupivacaine per hour suffices.

As has been described on p 123, lumbar epidural anesthesia can also be accomplished in children by means of an epidural catheter threaded up from the sacral hiatus.

Circulatory and respiratory complications with epidural or spinal blocks

Epidural or spinal blocks not only affect sensory and motor nerve fibers but also the sympathetic innervation of the peripheral vasculature, the heart (if extended to the T1 – T4 nerve roots), and visceral organs.

In epidural analgesia significant blood levels of the local anaesthetic and adrenaline are obtained which by themselves have direct effects on the heart as well as the peripheral vasculature. Clinically these effects add to a picture characterized by arterial hypotension but rarely bradycardia or respiratory disturbances. The magnitude of these complications is modified by patient-related factors such as cardiovascular disease, concomitant medication, and positive pressure ventilation.

A slight reduction of the arterial blood pressure should not be considered a complication of clinical significance. On the contrary, a moderate blood pressure reduction may in general be considered beneficial as cardiac work and thereby myocardial oxygen demand is reduced. Some degree of hypotension in relation to the preanesthetic value is therefore acceptable and should not require any therapy. In most patients a 20% reduction of mean arterial pressure can be considered safe, but elderly patients and patients with cardiovascular disease should be maintained closer to their normal blood pressure. A prerequisite for patient safety is that normal blood volume and adequate oxygenation are maintained and that the patient is kept in a horizontal or slightly head-down position.

The occurrence of yawning and mental confusion are definite warning signs of inadequate cerebral circulation secondary to arterial hypotension. The adequacy of myocardial perfusion, on the other hand, cannot be evaluated with certainty even when sophisticated monitoring is employed. As a consequence no general rules can be given as to the level of arterial hypotension that is safe in individual patients.

Falls in blood pressure secondary to these blocks can to some extent be prevented by avoiding too wide a distribution of block and by administration of a colloid (e.g., dextran 70, 300 – 500 ml) or crystalloid (1000 – 2000 ml) solution before and during the blockade, or, more effectively, by a vasopressor agent (e.g., ephedrine 25 – 50 mg or dihydroergotamine 0.5 – 1 mg) given subcutaneously prior to the blockade.

A more rational approach is to treat the hypotension when it comes. This can be done with small, sometimes repeated, doses of a vasopressor agent with alpha- as well as beta-adrenergic properties, such as ephedrine, 5 – 10 mg at a time, until a satisfactory blood pressure is obtained. Fluid therapy should be intensified at the same time, e.g., by rapid infusion of 500 ml dextran 70 or 1000 ml of Ringer's solution.

Respiration is generally unaffected by high spinal or epidural blocks per se. Sometimes patients experience dyspnea despite normal blood gases and unaffected ability to take a deep breath, probably due to decreased sensory input from proprioceptive nerve fibers in the chest wall.

Respiratory arrest is a classical feature of total spinal anesthesia. The cause is assumed to be arterial hypotension and ensuing brain stem ischemia and not blockade of the phrenic nerves. Treatment includes immediate endotracheal intubation, positive pressure ventilation until spontaneous respiration occurs, and measures against arterial hypotension.

Caudal (epidural) block

Epidural blockade can also be accomplished by the injection of a local anesthetic through the sacral hiatus, caudal block.

The anatomy of this area varies widely which must be kept in mind when performing this block. Ordinarily the two sacral cornu of the nonfused arch of the fifth sacral vertebra can be identified and the hiatus palpated between them, slightly cephalad in the midline.

The patient is placed in the prone position with a pillow under the hips. The table can in addition be flexed under the hips. The patient's legs are abducted and the feet inverted (Fig 2.30). The operator stands on the patient's left side and starts by identifying the midline of the sacrum and the angle between the sacrum and the coccyx. Slightly cephalad to the sacrococcygeal junction in the midline one should be able to identify one or two sacral cornu. After preparation of the skin the left thumb is placed between the cornu and is moved slightly cephalad, thereby stretching the skin and a wheal with local anesthetic raised. A 2.5- to 5-cm 23 or 25 gauge needle with a syringe containing local anesthetic is introduced at a 45° angle to the skin between the two cornu. No additional local anesthetic is injected as this will obscure the anatomy. The elastic resistance of the ligament covering the hiatus is gently sought for and when found the needle is advanced in approximately the same direction. If the needle is in the caudal epidural space it can be advanced a further 2 – 3 cm without any bone contact. After careful aspiration and with the finger of the free hand over the tip of the needle 3 – 5 cc of local anesthetic (or air) is injected rapidly. There should be no resistance to injection. If crepitation is felt or resistance occurs the needle is either in the subcutaneous tissue or subperiosteal.

It can sometimes be extremely difficult to localize the hiatus since the variations of the anatomy can be extreme. Caudal block, at least in adults, is one of the most unpredictable techniques, having varying

Fig. 2.30. Positioning of patient for caudal block.

Fig. 2.31. Testing of hypoalgesia within the S5 dermatome.

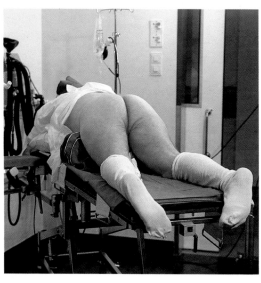

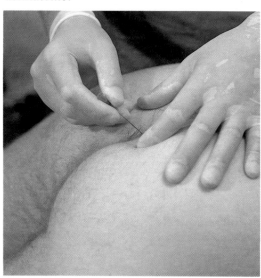

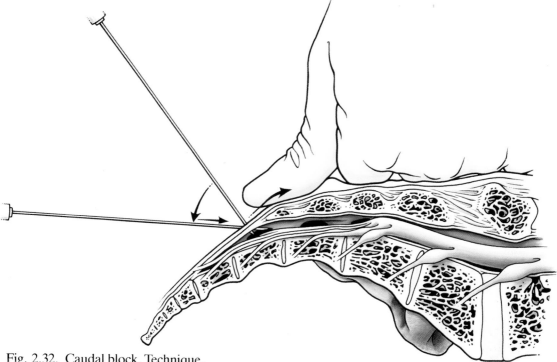

Fig. 2.32. Caudal block. Technique.

success rates. Even in the technically easy block, onset time, spread of analgesia, duration, etc are unreliable. In children however, caudal block is extremely easy to perform and produces quite satisfactory results.

As an aid to the evaluation of onset of block the following guidelines can be given:

1. For a successful block to ensue, definite hypoalgesia within the S5 dermatome should be present within 1 – 2 min after injection (Fig 2.31).

2. Likewise a definite reduction or disappearance of the anal sphincter reflex (contraction of the external sphincter secondary to pinprick of the perianal region) should be present at 4 – 5 min after injection.

3. The onset must be checked bilaterally as a unilateral block might result.

4. If signs 1 and 2 are not observed one should proceed with either a renewed attempt at caudal block, low spinal block, or general anesthesia.

Local anesthetic agents and doses

For adults an average of 20 ml of a solution of the short acting agents of the amide type is the standard. When long-lasting blocks are sought, 0.5% bupivacaine is used. It must be remembered that a caudal block frequently affects the ability to micturate and the motor power of the legs. The use of long-acting agents might therefore be the cause for insertion of a urinary bladder catheter or delaying full mobilization of patients postoperatively.

In children the dose is usually 0.1 ml/segment/year of age. By introducing a thin epidural catheter through a plastic cannula inserted in the hiatus, a continuous caudal block can be accomplished. In children the catheter can be introduced all the way up to the L1 level, thereby producing a lumbar epidural block.

123

Suggested reading

General

Abouleish E, Bourke D (1984) Concerning the use and abuse of test doses for epidural anesthesia. Anesthesiology 61:344

Abouleish E, Orig T, Amortequi AJ (1980) Bacteriologic comparison between epidural and caudal techniques. Anesthesiology 53:511

Abraham RA, Harris AP, Maxwell LG (1986) The efficacy of 1.5% lidocaine with 7.5% dextrose and epinephrine as an epidural test dose for obstetrics. Anesthesiology 64:116

Blomberg R (1985) A method for epiduroscopy and spinaloscopy. Presentation of preliminary results. Acta Anaesthesiol Scand 29:113

Bonica JJ (1954) Clinical evaluation of segmental peridural block. J Mich State Med Soc 53:167

Bromage PR (1962) Spread of analgetic solutions in the epidural space and their site of action. A statistical study. Br J Anaesth 34:161

Bromage PR (1965) A comparison of the hydrochloride and carbon dioxide salts of lidocaine and prilocaine in epidural analgesia. Acta Anaesthesiol Scand (Suppl) 16:55

Bromage PR (1975) Mechanism of action of extradural anaesthesia. Br J Anaesth 47:199

Bromage PR (1984) Current concepts and perspectives in epidural anaesthesia. In: van Kleef JW, Burm AGL, Spierdijk J (eds) Current concepts in regional anaesthesia. Proceedings of the second general meeting of the European Society of Regional Anaesthesia. Martinus Nijhoff, The Hague, p 151.

Bromage PR, Pettigrew RT, Crowell DE (1969) Tachyphylaxis in epidural analgesia: I. Augmentation and decay of local anesthesia. J Clin Pharmacol 9:30

Burn JM, Guyer PB, Langdon L (1973) The spread of solutions injected into the epidural space. A study using epidurograms in patients with the lumbosciatic syndrome. Br J Anaesth 45:338

Carrie LES (1971) The approach to the extradural space. Anaesthesia 26:252

Casey WF (1985) Epidural test doses in obstetrics. Anaesthesia 40:597

Cohen S, Luykx WM, Marx GF (1984) High versus low flow rates during lumbar epidural block. Reg Anesth 9:8

Cusick JF, Myklebust JB, Abram SE (1980) Differential neural effects of epidural anesthesia. Anesthesiology 53:299

Fink BR (1986) Mechanism of differential epidural block. Anesth Analg 65:325

Galindo A, Hernandez J, Benavides O et al. (1975) Quality of spinal extradural anaesthesia: the influence of spinal nerve root diameter. Br J Anaesth 47:41

Hilt H, Gramm H-J, Link J (1986) Changes in intracranial pressure associated with extradural anaesthesia. Br J Anaesth 58:676

Inoue R, Suganuma T, Echizen H et al. (1985) Plasma concentrations of lidocaine and its principal metabolites during intermittent epidural anesthesia. Anesthesiology 63:304

James FM, George RH, Naiem H et al. (1976) Bacteriologic aspects of epidural analgesia. Anesth Analg 55:187

McLeskey CH (1982) Identification of epidural space. Reg Anesth 7:171

Mehta M, Salmon N (1985) Extradural block. Confirmation of the injection site by X-ray monitoring. Anaesthesia 40:1009

Moore DC, Batra MS (1981) The components of an effective test dose prior to epidural block. Anesthesiology 55:693

Muneyuki M, Shirai K, Inamoto A (1970) Roentgenographic analysis of the positions of catheters in the epidural space. Anesthesiology 33:19

Murphy TM, Mather LE, Stanton-Hicks M d'A et al. (1976) The effects of adding adrenaline to etidocaine and lignocaine in extradural anaesthesia. I: Block characteristics and cardiovascular effects. Br J Anaesth 48:893

Nishimura N, Kitahara T, Kusakabe T (1959) The spread of lidocaine and I^{131} solution in the epidural space. Anesthesiology 20:785

Reisner LS (1976) Epidural test solution or spinal fluid? Anesthesiology 44:451

Renck H, Torbergsen T (1978) Unusual response to extra-dural analgesia in the presence of an intra-dural spinal tumour. Br J Anaesth 50:845

Shah JL (1984) Effect of posture on extradural pressure. Br J Anaesth 56:1373

Shanda TR, Evans JA (1972) The relationship of epidural anesthesia to neural membranes and arachnoid villi. Anesthesiology 37:543

Sharrock NE (1979) Recordings of, and an anatomical explanation for, false positive loss of resistance during lumbar extradural analgesia. Br J Anaesth 51:253.

Stonham J, Moss P (1983) The optimal test dose for epidural anesthesia. Anesthesiology 58:389

Usubiaga JE, Dos Reis Jr A, Usubiaga LE (1970) Epidural misplacement of catheters and mechanisms of unilateral blockade. Anesthesiology 32:158

Van Zundert A, Vaes L, van der Aa P et al (1986) Motor blockade during epidural anesthesia. Anesth Analg 65:333

Wildsmith JAW (1986) Editorial: extradural blockade and intracranial pressure. Br J Anaesth 58:579

Zarzur E (1984) Anatomic studies of the human lumbar ligamentum flavum. Anesth Analg 63:499

Dose requirements

Andersen S, Cold GE (1981) Dose response studies in elderly patients subjected to epidural analgesia. Acta Anaesthesiol Scand 25:278

Attia J, Sandouk P, Ecoffey C et al (1985) Pharmacokenitics following epidural morphine in children. Anesthesiology 63:A469

Bromage PR (1962) Exaggerated spread of epidural analgesia in arteriosclerotic patients. Br Med J 2:1634

Bromage PR (1969) Ageing and epidural dose requirements. Segmental spread and predictability of epidural analgesia in youth and extreme age. Br J Anaesth 41:1016

Bromage PR et al (1969) Tachyphylaxis in epidural analgesia; Augmentation and decay of local anaesthesia. J Clin Pharmacol 9:30

Grundy EM, Ramamurthy S, Patel KP et al. (1978) Extradural analgesia revisited. A statistical study. Br J Anaesth 50:805

Inoue R, Suganuma T, Echizen H et al (1985) Plasma concentrations of lidocaine and its principal metabolites during intermittent epidural anesthesia. Anesthesiology 63:304

Lanz E, Kehrberger E, Theiss E et al (1985) Epidural morphine: a clinical double-blind study of dosage. Anesth Analg 68:786

Lund C, Mogensen T, Hjortso NC et al (1985) Systemic morphine enhances spread of sensory analgesia during postoperative epidural bupivacaine infusion. Lancet ii:1156

Nickel PM, Bromage PR, Sherril DL (1986) Comparision of hydrochloride and carbonated salts of lidocaine for epidural analgesia. Reg Anesth 11:62

Nordberg G, Mellstrand T, Borg L et al (1986) Extradural morphine: Influence of adrenaline admixture. Br J Anaesth 58:598

Park WY, Massengale M, Kim SI et al (1980) Age and the spread of local anesthetic solutions in the epidural space. Anesth Analg 59:768

Park WY, Hagins FM, Rivat EL et al. (1982) Age and epidural dose response in adult men. Anesthesiology 56:318

Renck H (1980) Tachyphylaxis during postoperative peridural analgesia of long action. In: Wöst HJ, Zindler M (eds) Neue Aspekte in der Regionalanaesthesie 1.(Anaesthesiology and intensive care medicine vol 124) Springer, Berlin, pp 188 – 191.

Sharrok NE (1977) Lack of exaggerated spread of epidural anesthesia in patients with arteriosclerosis. Anesthesiology 47:307

Sharrock NE (1978) Epidural anesthetic dose responses in patients 20 to 80 years old. Anesthesiology 49:425

Sharrock NE, Lesser ML, Gabel RA (1984) Segmental levels of anaesthesia following the extradural injection of 0.75% bupivacaine at different lumbar spaces in elderly patients. Br J Anaesth 56:285

Tucker GT, Cooper S, Littlewood D et al. (1977) Observed and predicted accumulation of local anaesthetic agents during continuous epidural analgesia. Br J Anaesth 49:237

Usubiaga JE, Wikinski JA, Usubiaga LE (1967) Epidural pressure and its relation to spread of anesthetic solutions in epidural space. Anesth Analg 46:440

Thoracic epidural anesthesia

Bromage PR (1974) Lower limb reflex changes in segmental epidural analgesia. Br J Anaesth 46:504.

Reiz S, Häggmark S, Rydvall A et al. (1982) Beta-blockers and thoracic epidural analgesia. Cardioprotective and synergistic effects. Acta Anaesthesiol Scand (Suppl 4) 76:54

Renck H, Edström H (1975) Thoracic epidural analgesia I – a double blind study betweeen bupivacaine and etidocaine. Acta Anaesthesiol Scand (Suppl) 57:89

Renck H, Edström H, Kinnberger B et al. (1976) Thoracic epidural analgesia II – prolongation in the early postoperative period by continuous injection of 1.0% bupivacaine. Acta Anaesthesiol Scand 20:47.

Renck H, Edström H (1976) Thoracic epidural analgesia III – prolongation in the early postoperative period by intermittent injections of etidocaine with adrenaline. Acta Anaesthesiol Scand 20:104

Schulte-Steinberg O, Ostermayer R, Rahlts VW (1984) Thoracic epidural analgesia. Relationship between dose of etidocaine and spread of analgesia. Reg Anaesth 9:78

Caudal epidural anesthesia

Armitage EN (1979) Caudal block in children. Anaesthesia 34:396

Arthur DS (1980) Caudal anaesthesia in neonates and infants. Anaesthesia 35:1136

Busoni P, Andreuccetti T (1986) The spread of caudal analgesia in children: a mathematical model. Anaesth intens Care 14:140

Ecoffey C, Desparmet J, Maury M et al.(1985) Bupivacaine in children: pharmacokinetics following caudal anesthesia. Anesthesiology 63:447

Eyres RL, Hastings C, Brown TCK et al (1986) Plasma bupivacaine concentrations following lumbar epidural anaesthesia in children. Anaesth Intens Care 14:131

McGown RG (1982) Caudal analgesia in children. Five hundred cases for procedures below the diaphragm. Anaesthesia 37:806

Nolte H, Heege G, Hadinia A (1970) Indikationen und Möglichkeiten der Caudalanaesthesie unter Berücksichtigung des hohen Lebensalters. In: Hutschenreuter K, Bihler K, Fritsche P, (eds) Anaesthesie in extremen Altersklassen. (Anaesthesiology and Resuscitation, vol 47) Springer, Berlin, p 233.

Park WY, Massengale M, MacNamara RE (1979) Age, height and speed of injection as factors determining caudal anesthetic level, and occurrence of severe hypertension. Anesthesiology 51:81

Satoyoshi M, Kamiyama Y (1984) Caudal anaesthesia for upper abdominal surgery in infants and children: a simple calculation of the volume of local anaesthetic. Acta Anaesthesiol Scand 28:57

Schulte-Steinberg O, Rahlts VW (1970) Caudal anaesthesia in children and spread of 1 percent lignocaine. A statistical study. Br J Anaesth 42:1093

Schulte-Steinberg O, Rahlts VW (1977) Spread of extradural analgesia following caudal injection in children. A statistical study. Br J Anaesth 49:1027

Takasaki M (1984) Blood concentrations of lidocaine, mepivacaine and bupivacaine during caudal analgesia in children. Acta Anaesthesiol Scand 28:211

Takasaki M, Dohi S, Kawabata Y et al. (1977) Dosage of lidocaine for caudal anesthesia in infants and children. Anesthesiology 47:527

Warner MA, Kunkel SE, Dawson B et al (1985) The effects of age and addition of epinephrine to bupivacaine for caudal analgesia in pediatric patients. Anesthesiology 63:A464

Weber S (1985) Caudal anesthesia complicated by intraosseous injection in a patient with ankylosing spondylitis. Anesthesiology 63:716

Ventilatory/circulatory effects of epidural/spinal anesthesia

Arndt JO, Hock A, Stanton-Hicks M et al. (1985) Peridural anesthesia and the distribution of blood in supine humans. Anesthesiology 63:616

Baron J-F, Decaux-Jacolot A, Edouard A, Berdeaux A et al. (1986) Influence of venous return on baroreflex control of heart rate during lumbar epidural anesthesia in humans. Anesthesiology 64:188

Beardsworth D, Lind LJ (1985) Bladder distension and cardiovascular depression during recovery from epidural anesthesia. Reg Anesth 10:184

Bengtsson M (1984) Changes in skin blood flow and temperature during spinal analgesia evaluated by laser Doppler flowmetry and infrared thermography. Acta Anaesthesiol Scand 28:625

Bonica JJ, Berges PU, Morikawa K (1970) Circulatory effects of peridural block: I. Effects of level of analgesia and dose of lidocaine. Anesthesiology 33:619

Bonica JJ, Akamatsu T, Berges PU et al. (1971) Circulatory effects of peridural block: II. Effects of epinephrine. Anesthesiology 34:514

Bonica JJ, Kennedy WFjr, Akamatsu TJ et al. (1972) Circulatory effects of peridural block: III. Effects of acute blood loss. Anesthesiology 36:219

Castenfors J, Lindblad LE, Mortasawi A (1975) Effect of dihydroergotamine on peripheral circulation during epidural anaesthesia in man. Acta Anaesthesiol Scand 19:79.

Cousins MJ, Wright CJ (1971) Graft, muscle, skin blood flow after epidural block in vascular surgical procedures. Surg Gynec Obstet 133:59

Dohi S, Tsuchida H, Mayumi T (1983) Baroreflex control of heart rate during cardiac sympathectomy by epidural anesthesia in lightly anesthetized humans. Anesth Analg 62:815

Ecoffey C, Edouard A, Pruszcynski W, Taly E et al. (1985) Effects of epidural anesthesia on catecholamines, renin activity and vasopressin changes induced by tilt in elderly men. Anesthesiology 62:294

Engberg G (1977) The circulatory effects of ephedrine in connection with epidural analgesia. With special reference to the use of long-acting local anaesthetic agents Acta Universitatis Upsaliensis. Abstracts of Uppsala Dissertations from the Faculty of Medicine. 268

Engberg G, Wiklund L (1978) The circulatory effects of intravenously administered ephedrine during epidural blockade. Acta Anaesthesiol Scand 66:27

Germann PAS, Roberts JG, Prys-Roberts C (1979) The combination of general anaesthesia and epidural block. I: The effects of sequence of induction on haemodynamic variables and blood gas measurements in healthy patients. Anaesth Intensive Care 7:229

Green NM (1981) Physiology of spinal anesthesia, 3rd edn. Williams & Wilkins, Baltimore.
Green NM (1981) Preganglionic sympathetic blockade in man: a study of spinal anesthesia. Acta Anaesthesiol Scand 25:463

Kennedy WF Jr., Sawyer TK, Gerbershagen HU et al. (1976) Systemic cardiovascular and renal hemodynamic alterations during peridural anesthesia in normal man. Anesthesiology 31:414

Kety SS, King BD, Horvath SM et al. (1950) The effects of an acute reduction in blood pressure by means of differential sympathetic block on the cerebral circulation of hypertensive patients. J Clin Invest 29:402

Kleinerman J, Sancetta SM, Hackel DB (1958) Effects of high spinal anesthesia on cerebral circulation and metabolism in man. J Clin Invest 37:285

Lund R, Hedenstierna G, Johansson H (1983) Ventilation perfusion relationship during epidural analgesia. Acta Anaesthesiol Scand 27:410

Lynn RB, Sancetta SM, Simeone FA et al. (1952) Observations on the circulation in high spinal anesthesia. Surgery 32:195

Mattila M, Hannonen P, Puttonen E et al. (1985) Dihydroergotamine in the prevention of hypotension associated with extradural anaesthesia. Br J Anaesth 57:976

McCarthy GS (1976) The effect of thoracic epidural analgesia on pulmonary gas distribution, functional residual capacity and airway closure. Br J Anaesth 48:243

Nishimura N, Kajimoto Y, Kabe T et al (1985) The effects of volume loading during epidural analgesia. Resuscitation 13:31

Ottesen S (1978) The influence of thoracic epidural analgesia on the circulation at rest and during physical exercise in man. Acta Anaesthesiol Scand 22:537

Otton PE, Wilson EJ (1966) The cardiocirculatory effects of upper thoracic epidural analgesia. Can Anaesth Soc J 13:541

Reiz S, Nath S, Rais O (1980) Effects of thoracic epidural block on coronary vascular resistance and myocardial metabolism in patients with coronary artery disease. Acta Anaesthesiol Scand 24:11

Sjögren S, Wright B (1972) Circulatory changes during continuous epidural blockade. Acta Anaesthesiol Scand (Suppl) 46:5

Sjögren S, Wright B (1972) Respiratory changes during continuous epidural blockade. Acta Anaesthesiol Scand (Suppl) 46:27

Sundberg A, Wattwil M, Arvill A (1986) Respiratory effects of high thoracic epidural anaesthesia. Acta Anaesthesiol Scand 30:215

Takeshima R, Dohi S (1985) Circulatory responses to baroreflexes, valsalva maneuver, coughing, swallowing, and nasal stimulation during acute cardiac sympathectomy by epidural blockade in awake humans. Anesthesiology 63:500

Wahba WM, Don HF, Craig DB (1975) Post-operative epidural analgesia: effects on lung volumes. Can Anaesth Soc J 22:519

Wattwil M, Sundberg A, Arvill A et al. (1985) Circulatory changes during high thoracic epidural anaesthesia – influence of sympathetic block and of systemic effect of the local anaesthetic. Acta Anaesthesiol Scand 29:849

Wright GJ, Cousins MJ (1972) Blood flow distribution in the human leg following epidural sympathetic blockade. Arch Surg 105:334

Wöst HJ, Sandmann W, Florack G et al. (1980) Änderung der Hämodynamik während Regionalanaesthesie beim Hypertoniker. In: Wöst HJ, Zindler M (eds) Neue Aspekte in der Regionalanaesthesie 1. (Anaesthesiology and intensive care medicine, vol 124) Springer, Berlin. p 77

Complications of epidural anesthesia

Allemann BH, Gerber H, Gruber UH (1983) Rückenmarksnahe Anaesthesie und subkutan verabreichtes low-dose Heparin-Dihydergot zur Thromboembolieprophylaxe.Der Anaesthesist 32:80

Bromage PR (1985) Subdural migration of an epidural catheter. Anesth Analg 64:1029

Butler AB, Green CD (1970) Haematoma following epidural anaesthesia. Can Anaes Soc J 17:635

Cousins MJ (1972) Hematoma following epidural block. Anesthesiology 37:263

Crawford JS (1985) Some maternal complications of epidural analgesia for labor. Anaesthesia 40:1219

Crowhurst PE (1985) Accidental dural puncture. Anaesth Intens Care 13:213

Cucchiara RF, Wedel DJ (1984) Finding cerebrospinal fluid during epidural anesthesia. Anesth Analg 63:1121

DeAngelis J (1972) Hazards of subdural and epidural anesthesia during anticoagulant therapy: a case report and review. Anesth Analg 51:676

Evans JM, Gauci CA, Watkins G (1975) Horner's syndrome as a complication of lumbar epidural block. Anaesthesia 30:774

Gingrich TF (1968) Spinal epidural hematoma following continuous epidural anesthesia. Anesthesiology 29:162

Gissen AJ, Datta S, Lambert D (1984) The chloroprocaine controversy. I. A hypothesis to explain the neural complications of chloroprocaine epidural. Reg Anesth 9:124

Greensite FS, Katz J (1980) Spinal subdural hematoma associated with attempted epidural anesthesia and subsequent continuous spinal anesthesia. Anesth Analg 59:72

Harrison PD (1975) Paraplegia following epidural analgesia. Anaesthesia 30:778

Helne FW, Muechler HC (1965) Complications associated with the use of an extradural catheter in obstetric anesthesia. Anesth Analg 44:245

Helperin SW, Cohen DD (1971) Hematoma following epidural anesthesia: report of a case. Anesthesiology 35:641

Henderson JJ, MacRae WA (1983) Complications. In: Henderson JJ,Nimmo WS (eds) Practical regional anesthesia. Blackwell Scientific, Oxford, p 88

Hirsch NP, Child CS, Wijetilleka SA (1985) Paraplegia caused by spinal angioma – possible association with epidural analgesia. Anesth Analg 64:937

Hodgkinson R (1981) Total spinal block after epidural injection into an interspace adjacent to a dural perforation. Anesthesiology 55:593

Janis KM (1972) Epidural hematoma following postoperative epidural analgesia: a case report. Anesth Analg 51:689

Kancir CB, Petersen PH, Wandrup J (1985) Plasma magnesium during epidural anaesthesia. A study in patients undergoing transurethral prostatectomy. Anaesthesia 40:1165.

Kane RE (1981) Neurologic complications following epidural or spinal anesthesia. Anesth Analg 60:150

Kim YI, Mazza NM, Marx GF (1975) Massive spinal block with hemicranial palsy after a "test dose" for extradural analgesia. Anesthesiology 43:370

Kriz M, Joupilla R (1980) Subarachnoid block after a 'top-up' dose during continuous segmental epidural analgesia in labour. A case report. Acta Anaesthesiol Scand 24:495

Laman EN, McLeskey CH (1978) Supraclavicular subcutaneous emphysema following lumbar epidural anesthesia. Anesthesiology 48:219

Lanz E, Theiss D, Reiff K (1984) Seizure during repositioning following epidural anesthesia. Reg Anaesth 9:28

Massey Dawkins CJ (1969) An analysis of the complications of extradural and caudal block. Anaesthesia 24:554

McCullough JD, Stanley TH, Lunn JK (1980) Anticoagulants and continuous epidural anesthesia. Letter to the editor. Anesth Analg 59:394

McDonogh AJ, Cranney BS (1984) Delayed presentation of an epidural abscess. Anaesth Intens Care 12:364

Meyer HH, Mlasowsky B, Ziemer G et al (1985) Massive Blutung nach multiplen epiduralen Punktionen als Spätkomplikation bei Thrombozythämie.

Mohan J, Potter JM (1975) Pupillary constriction and ptosis following caudal epidural analgesia. Anaesthesia 30:769

Motsch J, Hutschenreuter K (1984) Cutane Liquorfistel im Anschluss an eine sekundäre Duraperforation durch einen Periduralkatheter. Reg Anaesth 7:74

Nash TG, Openshaw DJ (1968) Unusual complication of epidural anaesthesia. Br Med J II:700

Odoom JA, Sih IL (1983) Epidural analgesia and anticoagulant therapy. Experience with one thousand cases of continuous epidurals. Anaesthesia 38:254

Philip BK (1985) Effect of epidural air injection on catheter complications. Reg Anesth 10:21

Philip JH, Brown WU (1976) Total spinal anesthesia late in the course of obstetric bupivacaine epidural block. Anesthesiology 44:340

Pither CE, Hartrick CJ, Raj PP (1985) Heel sores in association with prolonged epidural analgesia. Anesthesiology 63:459

Plötz J, Schreiber W (1984) Intrazerebrale Massenblutung und Arteriaspinalis-anterior-Syndrom in ursächlichem Zusammenhang mit röckenmarksnahen Betäubungsverfahren? Zwei Fallbeschreibungen. Anästh Intensivther Notfallmed 19:307

Rainbird A, Pfitzner A (1983) Restricted spread of analgesia following epidural blood patch. Case report with a review of possible complications. Anaesthesia 38:481

Rao TLK, El-Etr AA (1981) Anticoagulation following placement of epidural and subarachnoidal catheters: an evaluation of neurologic sequelae. Anesthesiology 55:618

Ravindran R, Albrecht W, McKay M (1979) Apparent intravascular migration of epidural catheter. Anesth Analg 58:252

Rice P, Ethans CT (1986) Difficult removal of epidural catheters in the sitting position. Anesth Analg 65:539

Skouen JS, Wainapel SF, Willock MM (1985) Paraplegia following epidural anesthesia. A case report and a literature review. Acta NeurolScand 72:437

Stevens RA, Stanton-Hicks M (1985) Subdural injection of local anesthetic: a complication of epidural anesthesia. Anesthesiology 63:323

Tio TO, MacMurdo SD, McKenzie R (1979) Mishaps with an epidural catheter. Anesthesiology 50:260

Usubiaga JE (1975) Neurological complications following epidural anesthesia. Int Anesthesiol Clin 13:1

Vandam LD (1983) Complications of spinal and epidural anesthesia. In: Orkin FK, Cooperman LH, (eds) Complications in anesthesiology. J.B. Lippincott, Philadelphia, p 75.

Varke GP, Brindle GF (1974) Peridural anaesthesia and anti-coagulant therapy. Can Anaesth Soc J 21:106

Verniquet AJW (1980) Vessel puncture with epidural catheters. Experience in obstetric patients. Anaesthesia 35:660

Wanscher M, Riishede L, Krogh B (1985) Fistula formation following epidural catheter. A case report. Acta Anaesthesiol Scand 29:552

Wennigsted-Torgård K, Heyn J, Willumsen L (1982) Spondylitis following epidural morphine. Acta Anaesthesiol Scand 26:649

Zebrowski ME, Gutsche BB (1979) More on intravascular migration of an epidural catheter. Anesth Analg 58:531

126

Stellate ganglion block

The sympathetic preganglionic fibers to the head, neck, upper limb, and heart leave the spinal cord from segments T1 to T6 – T8. They converge to form the stellate ganglion, which may be divided into an inferior cervical and a first thoracic ganglion. It is located in a fascial plane limited posteriorly by the prevertebral fascia and anteriorly by the carotid sheath. The anatomy shows great individual variations, which explains the results obtained with stellate ganglion blockade.

Fig. 2.33. Stellate ganglion block. Technique, lateral view.

1. Cricoid cartilage
2. Stellate ganglion
3. Middle cervical ganglion
4. Transverse process of C6

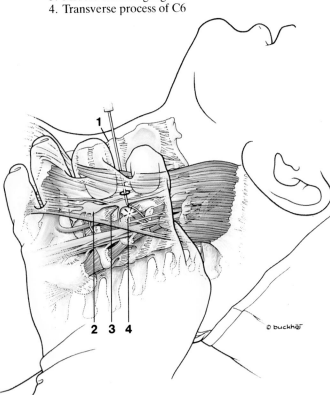

The patient is placed supine with a thin pillow under the neck and shoulders, so that the head is tilted slightly backward, and told to breath through the mouth (in order to relax the neck muscles). The second and third digits of the left hand are gently inserted between the trachea and the sternocleidomastoid muscle on the appropriate side at the C6 level, which is opposite the cricoid cartilage. The transverse process of vertebra C6 (Chassaignac's tubercle) is palpated. The two fingers, approximately 2 cm apart, are gently pressed down, pulling the carotid sheath laterally. A 3- to 5-cm 22 gauge block needle, attached to a 10-ml syringe filled with local anesthetic, is introduced between the two fingers perpendicular to the skin till it hits the transverse process. This usually occurs at a depth of 1 – 2 cm. The needle is then withdrawn 2 – 5 mm. With the needle firmly fixed, an aspiration test is performed and a test dose of 1 ml is injected if the aspiration test is negative. If no immediate signs of CNS toxicity follow the test dose, 6 – 10 ml is injected.

In order to accomplish a complete cervicothoracic sympathetic block the local anesthetic should fill the space ventral to the prevertebral fascia down to at least T4. This requires no cephalad spread (maintained pressure of the cephalad finger of the operator) and free caudad spread (release of pressure of the operator's caudad finger) of the local anesthetic. The neck is straightened and a larger pillow placed under the shoulders, neck, and head, elevating them about 15°. Occasionally higher doses, e.g., up to 15 ml, of the local anesthetic are necessary.

The occurrence of Horner's syndrome (ptosis, myosis, and endophthalmitis) indicates a successful block. Homolateral congestion of the nose, lack of sweating and hyperemia of the conjunctiva are other indications of a sympathetic block. These signs and symptoms might, however, be present without a complete sympathetic block of the arm.

Injection into the vertebral or carotid artery is a serious complication which immediately causes convulsions. If the injection takes place intradurally, spinal anesthesia ensues. Blockade of the recurrent laryngeal nerve, with resulting temporary hoarseness, is the commonest complication of the block which, for that reason, never should be performed bilaterally.

Neurolytic stellate ganglion block should rarely if ever be performed. Instead, thoracic sympathetic neurolysis at the appropriate levels should be considered.

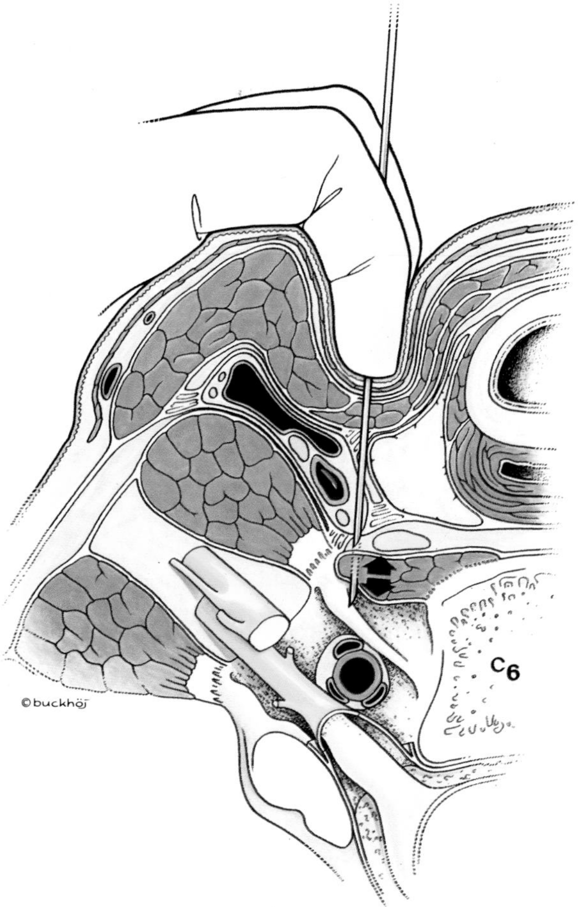

Suggested reading

Adriani J, Parmley J, Ochsner A (1952) Fatalities and complications after attempts at stellate ganglion block. Surgery 32:615

Allen G, Samson B (1986) Contralateral Horner's syndrome following stellate ganglion block. Can Anaesth Soc J 33:112

Boas RA (1981) The sympathetic nervous system and pain relief. In: Swerdlow M, (ed) Relief of intractable pain. Elsevier Scientific, Amsterdam, p 222

Boas RA, Hatangdi VS (1983) Chemical sympathectomy – techniques and responses. In: Yokota T, Dubner R (eds) Current topics in pain research and therapy. Proceedings of the international symposium on pain. Kyoto, Dec 12–13,1982. Excerpta Medica, Amsterdam, p 259

Fig. 2.34. Stellate ganglion block. Technique, cross section at the C6 level.

Fig. 2.35. Stellate ganglion block. Technique.

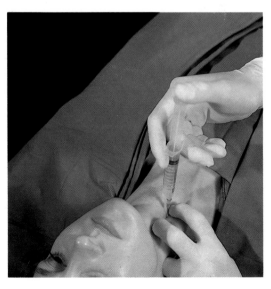

Thoracic Paravertebral Block

Although the patient can be placed in the lateral position for unilateral block, with the affected side up, and in the prone position for bilateral block, our preference is to use the prone position for both uni- and bilateral blocks.

The patient lies prone with a soft large pillow under his chest. The dorsal spine superior to the nerve to be blocked is identified and a skin wheal made approximately 3 cm lateral to it. This should be over the transverse process of the immediately inferior vertebra. A 70- to 100-mm 22 gauge needle is inserted 3 – 4 cm until the transverse process is contacted, withdrawn into the subcutaneous tissue, and then reinserted so as to go medial and inferior to it. At a point about 3 cm further in depth, a paresthesia of the thoracic nerve should be encountered. At this point 3 – 5 ml of a 2% solution of one of the short-acting amides or – for long-lasting blockade – 0.5% bupivacaine with adrenaline should be injected. If a paresthesia is not obtained as the needle is advanced it will come into contact with the posterior lateral border of the vertebra. The needle should then be withdrawn into the subcutaneous tissue and redirected slightly more caudad or cephalad. If several insertions of the needle fail to produce a paresthesia and the bone is continually contacted, the needle should be withdrawn about 1 cm from the periosteum and 8 – 10 ml of the selected local anesthetic infiltrated after frequent aspirations as the needle is withdrawn very slowly toward the subcutaneous tissue.

Radiologic confirmation of needle placement is a great aid in performing this block but for technical reasons it is difficult to obtain in the upper thoracic area. The proximity of the needle tip to the pleura, epidural, and intrathecal spaces necessitates the utmost delicacy in performing the procedure. In addition, since the intercostal nerve is contacted at its origin, it is possible to inject into a dural sleeve, resulting in a spinal anesthetic.

The authors do not generally subscribe to the injection of neurolytic solutions in this area. It is safer and simpler to perform neurolytic injections in the thoracic region in the subarachnoid space.

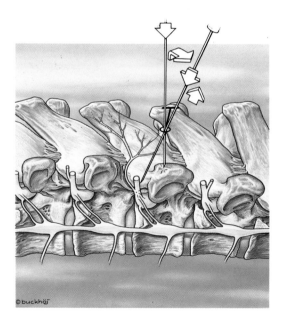

Fig. 2.36. Thoracic paravertebral block. Point of skin puncture and angulation of needle from position on the transverse process to position in relation to the spinal nerve just distal to the intervertebral foramen.

Thoracic Sympathetic Block

Since the upper thoracic ganglia lie in close proximity to the somatic nerves, they will almost always be blocked when a thoracic paravertebral somatic nerve block is successful. The technique for block of the upper ganglia is therefore the same as for thoracic paravertebral block. For the middle and lower thoracic ganglia, however, the needle should be advanced to the lateral aspect of the vertebral body.

For temporary blocks, 2 ml of a local anesthetic is injected at each ganglion. For permanent blocks (neurolysis), injection of a 6% – 10% phenol solution in a contrast medium is recommended. The spread of the solution, injected through a single needle, is visualized by fluoroscopy and the amount necessary to cover the appropriate ganglia is injected slowly under direct vision.

The danger of intrathecal injection can be minimized by the use of fluoroscopy. Pneumothorax may occur even several hours after the injection, so the patient should be hospitalized and kept under observation overnight.

Thoracic sympathetic blocks are followed by a greater incidence of complications than any other sympathetic block. In clinical practice thoracic sympathetic blocks can be replaced by either stellate ganglion block (p 128), for the upper thoracic sympathetic fibers, or by celiac plexus block, for the lower thoracic sympathetic fibers to the splanchnic area. Alternatively, segmental epidural blocks using small volumes of a dilute local anesthetic may be used in order to minimize the risk of complications.

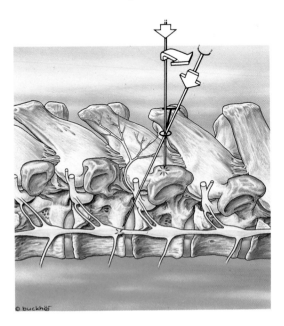

Fig. 2.37. Thoracic sympathetic ganglion block. Point of skin puncture and angulation of needle from position on the transverse process to the lateral aspect of the vertebral body.

131

Intercostal nerve block

Unilateral block

The patient is positioned semiprone with the side to be blocked uppermost. The patient's arm is raised above the head in order to lift the scapula away from the midline. The appropriate ribs are identified by counting up from the 12th rib.

Thumb and index fingers of the left hand bracket the rib at a point between the posterior axillary line and the costal angle, wherever the rib is easiest to palpate. A 25-mm 23 – 25 gauge needle (for the majority of patients) or a 50-mm 22 gauge needle (for the very muscular or obese) is used. The needle is directed at an angle of approximately 20° cephalad toward the rib (Fig 2.38a). The angle of the needle is maintained and the skin and needle are slowly moved in a caudad direction until the needle tip is felt to leave the rib at its caudad surface (Fig 2.38b). At this point the needle is advanced 2 – 3 mm (Fig 2.38c). Paresthesias are not sought. Between 3 and 5 cc of local anesthetic is injected after aspiration has ruled out an intravascular or intrapulmonary position of the needle tip by revealing no backflow of blood or air.

Bilateral block

The patient is placed in the prone position with both arms raised above the head (Fig 2.39). Generally the technique is then the same as for unilateral block. However, for practical purposes it is sometimes of benefit to modify the technique slightly. A patient under general anesthesia who is to undergo bilateral block cannot be placed in the prone position without considerable effort on the part of several people. With the aid of only one person the anesthesiologist can turn the patient 45° prone and perform bilateral blocks with the patient thus positioned (Fig 2.40).

Many anesthesiologists have performed intercostal blocks at the midaxillary line employing the same technique and dosage regimen as described above. An obvious advantage of this approach is the much easier access to the site of the block. In one small postoperative study the effectiveness of blocks performed in the midaxillary line was found to be equal to that of posterior intercostal blocks.

Fig. 2.38a–c. Intercostal nerve block. Technique.

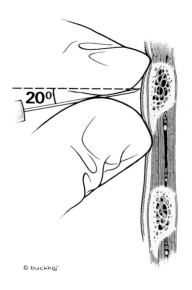
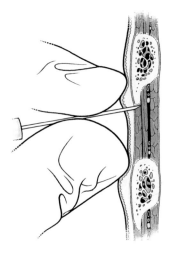
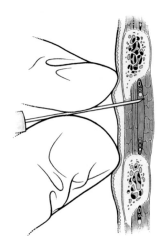

© buckhöj

Distribution and duration of block

Due to the overlapping innervation of the intercostal nerves a minimum of three nerves must be blocked in order to accomplish full analgesia of one segment. As described on p. 29 an overlap between the two sides exists, so for procedures which require midline incisions, bilateral nerve blocks must be performed.

From the above follows that a multitude of intercostal blocks are required for procedures through midline incisions. Since intercostal block is the nerve block procedure that is followed by the highest plasma concentrations of local anesthetic per milligram administered, a risk of overdosage exists. In order to avoid toxic symptoms the individual maximum dosage should always be calculated and never exceeded. In clinical practice 0.5% bupivacaine is almost exclusively used since this solution is long-acting and exerts only a moderate degree of motor blockade. Using 3 – 5 ml per intercostal nerve an average duration of sensory block of 4 – 5 hours is obtained. However, variations between 2 and almost 24 hours have been observed. The duration of block will not increase if larger doses per intercostal nerve is used. There is an obvious discrepancy between the duration of sensory block, as noted by reaction to pin-prick, versus freedom of pain in patients operated upon. For example around 75% of patients undergoing cholecystectomy require only one set of intercostal blocks for postoperative analgesia while reaction to pin-prick reappears after 4 – 8 hours.

In order to obtain prolonged pain relief by intercostal blocks either repetitive blocks or continuous techniques must be used. For the comfort of the patient, repetitive blocks should be performed before the effect of the preceding one has worn off. Continuous techniques by catheters inserted in a single or several intercostal space(s) have been tried. The position of multiple catheters is difficult to maintain from a practical point of view. The single catheter technique, however, results in adequate blockade of only one intercostal

Fig. 2.39. Intercostal nerve block. Prone positioning of patient.

Fig. 2.40. Intercostal nerve block. 45° prone positioning of patient for bilateral blocks.

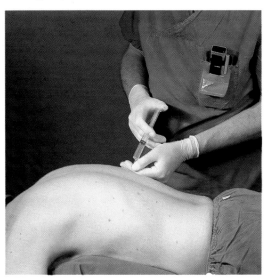

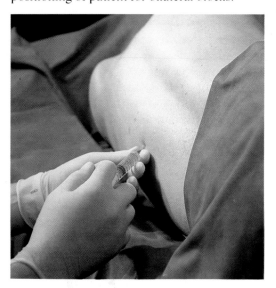

nerve. An important exception might be in patients with multiple rib fractures where the local anesthetic perhaps spreads in the fracture hematoma.

There is always the potential risk of pleural puncture and pneumothorax. However, the incidence seems to be extremely low even in inexperienced hands. When blocks are performed prior to or under general anesthesia employing positive pressure ventilation and nitrous oxide the risk of tension pneumothorax should always be kept in mind if circulatory or ventilatory complications occur.

Neurolytic blocks of intercostal nerves are associated with a high incidence of neuritis and should in general be replaced by subarachnoid neurolysis. In exceptional cases 1 ml of a 6% solution of phenol in water may be used. Because of the dermatomal overlap, a minimum of three nerves should be blocked.

Intercostal blocks by an intrapleural catheter technique.

This recently developed technique permits prolonged unilateral pain relief within an area supplied by the intercostal nerves. Clinical experience is very limited as yet and therefore only a brief description of the method is given.

With the patient lying on the contralateral side a 16 gauge Touhy needle is introduced at an angle of 30–40° in an appropriate intercostal space at the costal angle. The bevel of the needle is directed cephalad. After perforating the caudal intercostal membrane, which can be identified by its distinctive resistance to advancement of the needle, the stylet of the Touhy needle is removed and a well-lubricated air-filled all-glass syringe is attached to the needle hub. The syringe and needle are then carefully advanced. Puncture of the parietal pleura is noted by a "clicking" sensation in combination with a descent of the plunger as the negative intrapleural pres-

sure empties the air out of the syringe. After disconnection of the syringe an epidural catheter is threaded 5–6 cm into the pleural space and the needle is withdrawn. The catheter is trapped to the skin in the same way as in epidural anesthesia.

Twenty milliliters of 0.5% bupivacaine with adrenaline results in analgesia for approximately 9 hours (range 5–26 hours). Repeat doses of 20 ml are reported to result in analgesia for on average 11 hours. Continuous infusion of (0.25–) 0.5% bupivacaine, 5–10 ml/h, produces unilateral analgesia to 8–10 dermatomes. Plasma levels of local anaesthetics are reported to be lower with this method than with conventional intercostal blocks.

The method has been applied for postoperative analgesia, multiple rib fractures and acute thoracic herpes zoster. Its main advantage over conventional intercostal blocks is the accomplishment of multiple intercostal blocks over a prolonged period with only one skin puncture. The main advantage over continuous epidural blocks is the absence of motor block in the legs and of extensive sympathetic blockade with its related circulatory complications. Pneumothorax is a potential serious risk that so far has not been reported. Presently, the main indication for intrapleural block seems to be rib fractures in combination with pneumothorax requiring a chest drain. Only further experience with the method will reveal its place in the treatment of postoperative pain or pain secondary to pleuritis, herpes zoster, etc.

Suggested reading

Braid DP, Scott DB (1966) Effect of adrenaline: effect on the systemic vascular absorption of local anaesthetic drugs. Acta Anaesthesiol Scand (Suppl) 23:334

Bridenbaugh PO (1975) Intercostal nerve blockade for evaluation of local anaesthetic agents. Br J Anaesth 47:306

Brodsky JB (1979) Hypotension from intraoperative intercostal nerve blocks. Reg Anesth 4:17

Cottrell WM (1978) Hemodynamic changes after intercostal nerve block with bupivacaine- epinephrine solution. Anesth Analg 57:492

Jakobsson S (1977) Intercostal nerve blocks and chest wall mechanics. Abstracts of Uppsala Dissertations from the Faculty of Medicine 270

Johansson A, Renck H, Aspelin P et al. (1985) Multiple intercostal blocks by a single injection? A clinical and radiological investigation. Acta Anaesthesiol Scand 29:524

Moore DC (1981) Intercostal nerve block: spread of india ink injected to the ribs costal groove. Br J Anaesth 53:325

Moore DC, Mather LE, Bridenaugh LD et al. (1976) Arterial and venous plasma levels of bupivacaine following peripheral nerve blocks. Anesth Analg 55:763

Moore DC, Mather LE, Bridenbaugh PO et al. (1976) Arterial and venous plasma levels of bupivacaine following epidural and intercostal nerve blocks. Anesthesiology 45:39

Moore DC, Mather LE, Bridenbaugh LD et al. (1977) Bupivacaine (Marcaine): an evaluation of its tissue and systemic toxicity in humans. Acta Anaesthesiol Scand 21:109

Moore DC, Thompson GE, Crawford RD (1982) Long-acting local anesthetic drugs and convulsions with hypoxia and acidosis. Anesthesiology 56:230

Mulroy MF (1985) Intercostal block at the mid-axillary line. Reg Anesth 10:39

Murphy DF (1984) Continuous intercostal nerve blockade. Br J Anaesth 56:627

Murphy DF (1984) A new method of continuous intercostal nerve blockade: clinical and anatomical studies. Br J Anaesth 56:425

Nunn JF, Slavin G (1980) Posterior intercostal nerve block for pain relief after cholecystectomy. Anatomical basis and efficacy. Br J Anaesth 52:253

Pontén J, Biber B, Henriksson B-Å et al. (1982) Bupivacaine for intercostal nerve blockade in patients on long-term beta-receptor blocking therapy. Acta Anaesthesiol Scand (Suppl) 76:70

Reiestad F, Strömskag KE (1986) Interpleural catheter in the management of postoperative pain. A preliminary report. Reg Anesth 11:89

Rothstein P, Arthur GR, Feldman H et al. (1982) Pharmacokinetics of bupivacaine in children following intercostal block. Anesthesiology 57:A426

Scott DB (1965) Plasma levels of lignocaine (Xylocaine) and prilocaine (Citanest) following epidural and intercostal nerve block. Acta Anaesthesiol Scand (Suppl) 16:111

Telivou L, Perttala Y (1966) Use of x-ray contrast medium to control intercostal nerve blocks. Ann Chir Gynaecol 55:185

Willdeck-Lund G, Edström H (1975) Etidocaine in intercostal nerve block for pain relief after thoracotomy: a comparison with bupivacaine. Acta Anaesthesiol Scand (Suppl) 60:33

Block of the breast

Block of the breast is best accomplished by performing blocks of the third through seventh intercostal nerves using a total of 20 ml 0.5% bupivacaine with adrenaline, and infiltration of 10 – 15 ml 0.125% – 0.25% bupivacaine with adrenaline along the superior margin of the breast to block some superficial branches from the cervical plexus. If the breast is particularly pendulous or the skin incision extends below the seventh dermatome, additional infiltration of the line of skin incision is required.

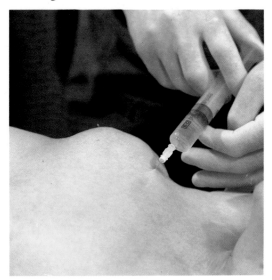

Fig. 2.41. Block of the breast. Subcutaneous infiltration of a local anesthetic along the superior margin of the breast.

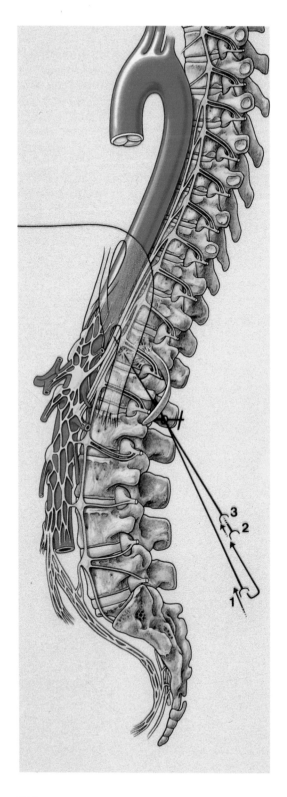

Splanchnic nerve block

The patient lies either prone over a small pillow placed under the upper abdomen (Fig. 2.43) or in the lateral position (Fig 2.45). At a point 5-7 cm lateral to the midline and just under the margin of the lowest rib a skin wheal is made. A transverse line drawn from this point to the dorsal spines usually bisects the L1 vertebra (Fig 2.46). However, due to variations of angulation of the twelth rib or its absence or shortness this method for the identification of the correct vertebral level is insecure and should be replaced by radiological identification. A 10-15-cm 22 gauge needle is inserted so as to contact the transverse process of L1. This should be at a depth of 3 – 5 cm. The needle is then withdrawn and redirected superiorly and medially to come into contact with the lateral aspect of the body of the T12 vertebra. The needle is then redirected and advanced to the anterior lateral sur-

Fig. 2.42. Splanchnic nerve block. Anatomy.

Fig. 2.43. Splanchnic nerve block. Prone position of patient.

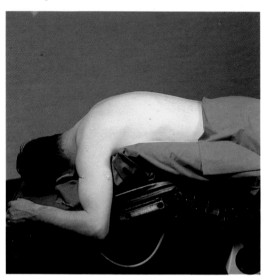

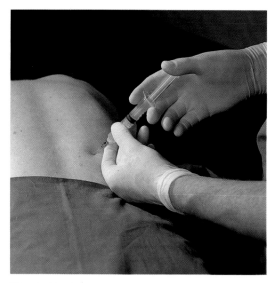

Fig. 2.44. Splanchnic nerve block. Technique of injection of patient in prone position.

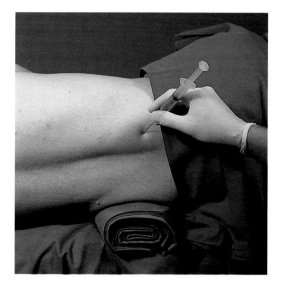

Fig. 2.45. Splanchnic nerve block. Technique of injection of patient in lateral position.

Fig. 2.46. Anatomical landmarks for splanchnic nerve block.

face of the vertebral body, where the nerves lie. Between 8 and 10 ml of a local anesthetic will block the splanchnic nerves.

Note

1. This procedure must be performed bilaterally to ensure optimal efficacy.

2. Advancement of the needle is more precise when using an image intensifier.

3. For almost all indications similar results can be obtained with celiac plexus block.

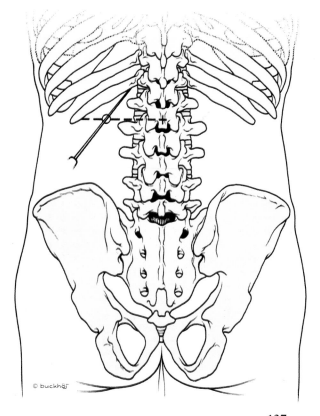

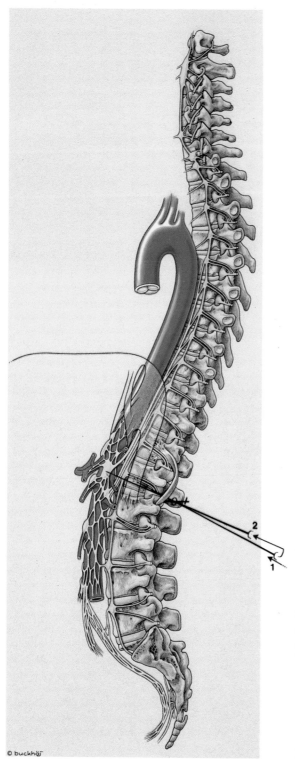

Celiac plexus block

Celiac plexus block is best done under fluoroscopic control to verify the position of the tip of the needle.

The patient lies prone with his head resting on a small pillow. Arms are abducted to slightly greater than 90° and bent at the elbows so that the patient is in a comfortable position.

The inferior border of the left twelfth rib is outlined and the dorsal spine of L1 identified. At a point 5 – 7 cm lateral to the inferior margin of the L1 spine and just beneath the lower border of the twelfth rib a 10- to 12-cm 22 gauge block needle is inserted at an angle of 30–45° toward the body of the L1 vertebra. The path through which the needle is to go should be generously infiltrated with local anesthetic. The needle is advanced until bone is met. If this occurs 3 – 5 cm below the skin, the transverse process has been contacted. The needle is then directed to pass either superiorly or inferiorly to the transverse process toward the body of the L1 vertebra. Contact with the body of the vertebra should preferably be confirmed by fluoroscopy. The angle of the needle is then reduced so that its tip passes just lateral to the margin of the body of L1. The needle is then guided approximately 2 – 3 cm past the lateral edge of the vertebra, at which point it should lie 1–2 cm deep to the anterior surface of the vertebral body. X-rays should verify this position. After careful aspiration to ascertain that the needle has not inadvertently entered the aorta or other major vessels a total of 30- 50 cc of a dilute local anesthetic solution, i.e., 0.25% bupivacaine, is injected.

Fig. 2.47. Celiac plexus block. Anatomy.

This block may be performed from either side but the left side is preferable since on the right the vena cava becomes another major vascular structure which should be avoided. (The vena cava runs just to the right of the midline in the area where the block is to be performed.) The block may also be performed with the patient in the lateral position. It is almost never necessary to perform the diagnostic block bilaterally when local anesthetics are used. In addition to vascular absorption one must be aware that significant postural hypotension frequently occurs following this block. Hypotension might be prevented or treated by volume replacement and/or the use of vasopressors.

Celiac plexus block with alcohol for prolonged pain relief is described on p 89.

Suggested reading

Boas RA (1978) Sympathetic blocks in clinical practice. Int Anesthesiol Clin 16:149

Boas RA, Hatangdi VS (1983) Chemical sympathectomy – techniques and responses. In: Yokota T, Dubner R (eds) Current topics in pain research and therapy. Proceedings of the international symposium on pain. Kyoto, Dec 12–13, 1982. Excerpta Medica, Amsterdam, p. 259.

Bonica J (1953) The management of pain. Lea and Febiger, Philadelphia, p.446.

Cherry DA, Rao DM (1982) Lumbar sympathetic and coeliac plexus blocks. An anatomical study in cadavers. Br J Anaesth 54:1037

De Sousa-Pereira A (1946) Blocking of the splanchnic nerves and the first lumbar sympathetic ganglion: technique, accidents and clinical indications. Arch Surg 53:32

Filshie J, Golding S, Robbie DS et al. (1983) Unilateral computerised tomography guided coeliac plexus block: a technique for pain relief. Anaesthesia 38:498

Fine PG, Bubela C (1985) Chylothorax following celiac plexus block. Anesthesiology 3:454

Jackson SH, Jacobs JB, Epstein RA (1969) A radiographic approach to coeliac plexus block. Anesthesiology 31:373

Moore DC, Bush WH, Burnett LL (1981) Celiac plexus block: a roentgenographic, anatomic study of technique and spread of solution in patients and corpses. Anesth Analg 60:369

Singler RC (1982) An improved technique for alcohol neurolysis of the celiac plexus. Anesthesiology 56:137

Ward EM, Rorie DK, Naus LA et al. (1979) The celiac ganglia in man: normal anatomic variations. Anesth Analg 58:461

Fig. 2.48. Celiac plexus block. Technique. The needles are introduced to pass transcrurally to ensure injection in the peri- and preaortal space. If the insertion of needles is made too laterally, there is a risk for injury of the kidney or renal pelvis.

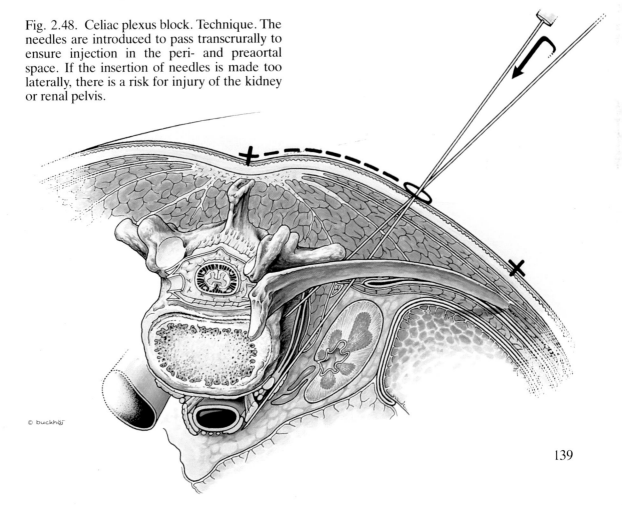

© buckhöj

139

Lumbar paravertebral block

The patient lies on his side opposite the one to be blocked. The correct vertebra of the nerve to be blocked is identified by counting either from L1 and/or from L4.

A skin wheal is made 3 – 5 cm lateral to the caudad tip of the appropriate dorsal spine. A 7- to 10-cm 22 gauge block needle is inserted perpendicular to the skin after infiltration of local anesthetic. The transverse process of the vertebra immediately below is contacted at a depth of 3 – 4 cm. The needle is then withdrawn and reinserted so as to pass just superior to the transverse process and in a slightly medial direction. At an additional depth of about 3 cm a paresthesia should be elicited. If it is not, the needle should be reinserted several times until a paresthesia is obtained. If attempts at paresthesias prove unsuccessful, the needle is advanced an additional 1 – 2 cm until it hits the lateral posterior border of the vertebral body at a depth of approximately 6- 8 cm from the skin. After withdrawal of the needle 0.5 – 1 cm from bone contact, infiltration of 8 – 10 ml of local anesthetic is made as the needle is moved in several directions. When a paresthesia is obtained, 5 ml will suffice for an adequate block to ensue.

When neurolytic agents are to be used the obtaining of paresthesias is mandatory. The procedure should be done with fluoroscopic verification of needle tip placement. Alternatively, a nerve stimulator can be used for optimal positioning of the needle in relation to the nerve.

If the block is to be done bilaterally the patient is best positioned prone and with a soft pillow placed underneath the abdomen. The procedure is then carried out exactly as described above.

It is important to remember that subarachnoid puncture is not infrequently obtained when performing these blocks, especially if paresthesias are difficult to obtain. If a large dose of the local anesthetic is injected a total spinal block may result.

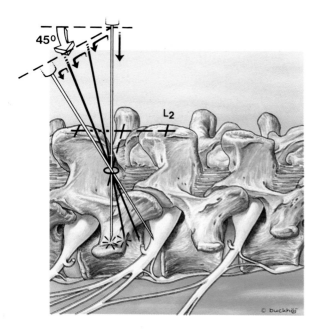

Fig. 2.49. Lumbar paravertebral block. Point of skin puncture and angulation of needle from position on the transverse process to position just lateral to the intervertebral foramen.

Transsacral block

The patient is placed in the prone position with a pillow under his hips. After skin preparation the most posterior and medial part of the iliac crest on the appropriate side is palpated. The second sacral foramen is located 1 cm medial and 1 cm caudad to this point. In order to localize the other posterior foramina of the sacrum, a line is drawn between this point and a point 1 cm lateral and 1 cm superior to the sacral cornu on the same side. This point overlies the fourth sacral foramen. The first sacral foramen is 2 cm above the second and the third is midway between the second and fourth.

For individual blocks of the sacral nerves, 22 gauge needles are introduced through skin wheals made at the above described places. The needle is introduced slightly medially and inferiorly to the perpendicular plane. The needle is advanced carefully until it hits the posterior surface of the sacrum. The depth is noted. The needle is slightly withdrawn and reinserted in a fanwise manner until it can be felt to pass into the foramen.

After careful aspiration a long-acting local anesthetic, such as 0.5% bupivacaine with adrenaline, is injected using 3–5 ml per nerve. Neurolytic agents could be used, e.g., 6% phenol in water.

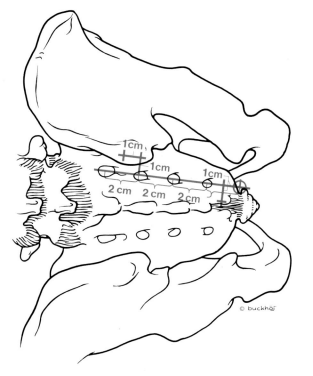

Fig. 2.50. Transsacral block. Identification of points of skin puncture.

141

Lumbar sympathetic block

Although this block may be performed using bony landmarks as the sole guide for needle position, fluoroscopic confirmation is recommended especially when performing neurolytic blocks.

The patient lies in the lateral position with the side to be blocked uppermost. The dorsal spine of L2 is identified by counting down from L1 or up from L4. The correct level is confirmed radiologically.

A 10- to 15-cm 22 gauge block needle is used, the choice depending upon the size of the patient. A skin wheal is raised 5 – 7 cm lateral to the caudal tip of the L2 spinous process. The soft tissue along the line that the needle will traverse is generously infiltrated with local anesthetic. The needle is inserted through the skin at an angle of approximately 30° toward the body of the vertebra. If the transverse process of the vertebra is encountered, which

A 5-ml air-filled syringe with a freely movable barrel is attached and gentle ballottement applied as the needle is advanced through the paravertebral muscle mass. There will be a slight resistance to the plunger until the needle penetrates the psoas fascia into the groove between the muscle and the vertebrae where the sympathetic ganglia lie.

Further fluoroscopic confirmation that the tip of the needle is at the anterior lateral surface of the vertebra should be obtained at this time. In addition injection of 0.5 – 1 ml of a radio-opaque material will show a characteristic linear spread if the needle is correctly positioned. If a patchy distribution occurs this indicates that the needle is still in the muscle mass and should be repositioned. Alternatively, the injection of 1 – 2 ml of air will reveal a corresponding distribution of a negative contrast but this can only be obtained with fluoroscopic equipment with a high resolution. Once a correct needle position is accomplished, 8 – 10 ml of a local anesthetic is injected.

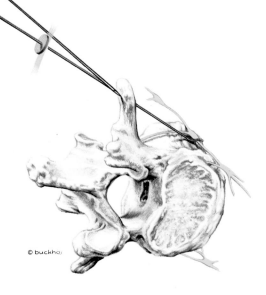

usually occurs at a depth of 3 – 5 cm, the needle should be redirected slightly cephalad or caudad. Once past the transverse process the needle is further advanced until the body of the vertebra is met, and this is preferably verified by fluoroscopy in two planes. The angle of the needle is then reduced so as to allow the needle tip to pass closely the lateral surface of the vertebra.

Fig. 2.51. Lumbar sympathetic block. Anatomy and technique.

© buckho;

Note: If neurolytic agents are to be injected the amount needed should be determined by watching the spread of the neurolytic agent (5% – 10% phenol dissolved in a radio-opaque substance). The dye should spread three vertebral bodies to ensure adequate interruption of the sympathetic chain. Careful aspiration should always be performed prior to injection of local anesthetics or neurolytic agents since the needle tip is very close to large vascular structures.

The risk of anaphylactic reactions to X-ray contrast media is always present, so adequate resuscitation equipment should be available at all times.

Suggested reading

Boas RA, Hatangdi VS (1983) Chemical sympathectomy – techniques and responses. In: Yokota T, Dubner R (eds) Current topics in pain research and therapy. Proceedings of the international symposium on pain, Kyoto, December 12–13, 1982. Excerpta Medica, Amsterdam, p 259

Brown EM, Kunjappan V (1975) Single-needle lateral approach for lumbar sympathetic block. Anesth Analg 54:725

Cherry DA (1978) A technical aid for the performance of neurolytic lumbar sympathectomy. Anaesth Intensive Care 6:164

Cherry DA, Rao DM (1982) Lumbar sympathetic and coeliac plexus blocks. An anatomical study in cadavers. Br J Anaesth 54:1037

Collins GJ, Rich NM, Andersen CA et al. (1978) Acute hemodynamic effects of lumbar sympathectomy. Am J Surg 136:714

Dam W (1962) Blokadebehandling. Nord Med 68:1098
Hatangdi VS, Boas RA (1985) Lumbar sympathectomy: a single needle technique. Br J Anaesth 57:285

Hughes-Davies DI, Redman LR (1976) Chemical lumbar sympathectomy. Anaesthesia 31:1068

Lundskog O, Baar HA, Ahlgren I (1973) 10 Jahre Erfahrung mit der Blockadetherapie. Anaesthesiol Wiederbelebung 73:27

Redman DRO, Robinson PN, Al-Kutoubi MA (1986) Computerised tomography guided lumbar sympathectomy. Anaesthesia 41:39

Fig. 2.52. Lumbar sympathetic block. Landmarks and direction of needle insertion.

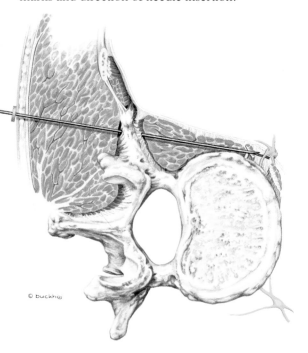

Fig. 2.53. Lumbar sympathetic block. Anatomy and technique.

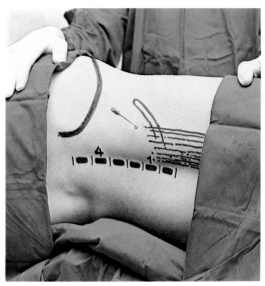

Block of the ilioinguinal and iliohypogastric nerves

The patient lies supine and the anterior superior iliac spine is identified. Approximately 2–3 cm from the spine, on a line between it and the umbilicus, a 5-cm 25 gauge block needle (in the average size adult) is inserted perpendicular to the skin. A slight "giving" sensation is noted when the needle pierces the external oblique muscle. Up to 10 ml of local anesthetic, e.g., 1% lidocaine or 0.25% bupivacaine, is then fanned along the most lateral part of the previously determined line from the anterior superior iliac spine to the umbilicus deep to the external oblique muscle. The needle should also be advanced slightly so as to pierce the internal oblique muscle to assure adequate block of the ilioinguinal nerve. Paresthesias are not sought.

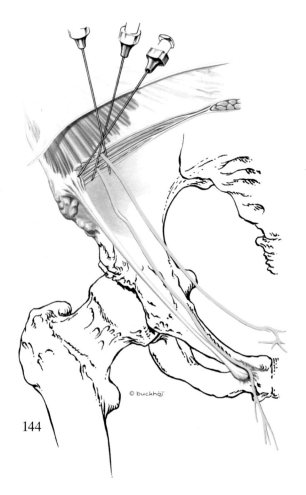

Fig. 2.54. Block of the ilioinguinal and iliohypogastric nerves.

144

Field block of the inguinal region

The ilioinguinal and iliohypogastric nerves are blocked as described in the preceding section. A 10-cm 25 gauge block needle is then advanced in the subcutaneous tissue, spreading local anesthetic from the iliac crest to the umbilicus. Twenty milliliters of a dilute local anesthetic is required to raise a skin wheal and infiltrate the deeper soft tissue layers. A second skin wheal is then raised from the iliac crest to the lateral aspect of the pubic tubercle. In addition 3 – 5 ml of local anesthetic is placed along the superior ramus of the pubis in order to anesthetize some terminal fibers of the genito-femoral nerve. It will be necessary for the operator to infiltrate the internal hernia ring to block the autonomic fibers that will be stimulated when the hernia sac is dissected and stretched.

Suggested reading

Ponka JL (1963) Seven steps to local anaesthesia for inguinofemoral hernia repair. Surg Gynecol Obstet 117:115

Fig. 2.55. Anatomy of the inguinal region.

1. Aponeurosis of the external oblique m.
2. External oblique m.
3. Internal oblique m.
4. Anterior superior iliac spine
5. Transversus abdominis m.
6. Iliohypogastric n.
7. Inguinal ligament
8. Ilioinguinal n.
9. Genital branch of the genitofemoral n.
10. Spermatic cord
11. Pubic tubercle
12. Superficial inguinal ring
13. Inguinal hernia

Fig. 2.56. Field block of the inguinal region.

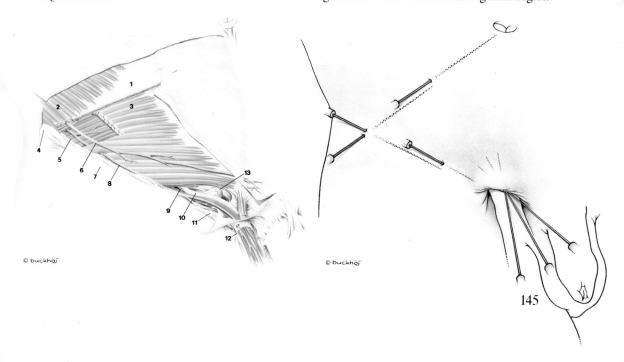

© buckhöj

© buckhöj

Upper abdominal field block

Skin wheals are raised at the tip of the xiphoid process of the sternum and the ends of the eighth, ninth, tenth, and eleventh ribs. A subcutaneous infiltration is carried out to connect the wheals. Through the wheals a 1- to 5-cm needle (the choice depending upon the size of the subcutaneous fat pad) is inserted and local anesthetic spread in a fanwise direction toward the parietal peritoneum. If the operation is limited to one side of the body, infiltration from the tip of the xiphoid to the umbilicus will eliminate the necessity of performing blocks on both sides. In addition to the above it is sometimes necessary to infiltrate local anesthesia directly over the incision site.

Note: Intercostal blocks, T6 through T10, provide the same degree of anesthesia as described above.

Fig. 2.57a. Upper abdominal field block. Technique.

Fig. 2.57b.

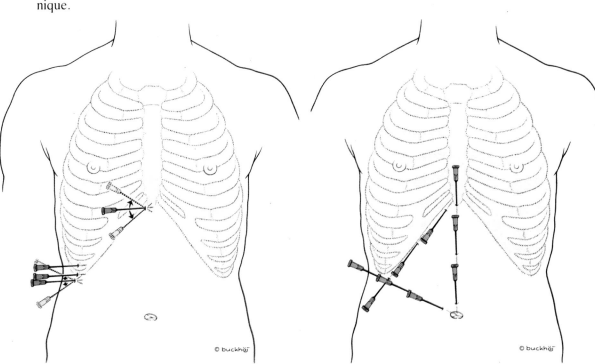

Obturator nerve block

The patient lies supine with the legs slightly spread. The spine of the pubic bone on the involved side is identified and a skin wheal made 3 cm lateral and inferior to the spine. After generous infiltration with local anesthetic a 7 cm 22 gauge block needle is inserted perpendicular to the skin wheal until the upper part of the inferior ramus of the pubic bone is contacted. This should be at a depth of 1 – 3 cm. The needle is then redirected so as to slip past the inferior ramus and just underneath the superior ramus of the pubic bone and advanced an additional 3 – 4 cm. This needle direction is lateral and slightly inferior. Paresthesias are usually not obtained although occasionally they may be found. Between 10 and 15 cc of local anesthetic is infiltrated into the area of the obturator foramen (which is where the needle tip should lie) as the needle is moved back and forth slowly.

A nerve stimulator can be of great aid when performing this block.

Suggested reading

Hradec E, Soukup F, Nova'k J et al (1983) The obturator nerve block. Preventing damage of the bladder wall during transurethral surgery. Int Urol Nephrol 15:149

Magora F, Rozin R, Ben-Menachem Y, et al (1969) Obturator nerve block: an evaluation of technique. Br J Anaesth 41:695

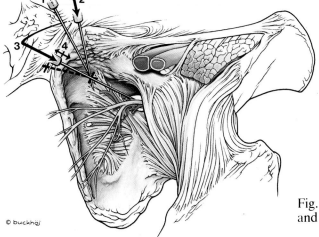

© buckhoj

Fig. 2.58. Obturator nerve block. Anatomy and technique.

Penile block

A 23 – 25 gauge needle is inserted just below the lower border of the pubic arch and advanced to the root of the penis, piercing Buck's fascia. Two-thirds of the local anesthetic is injected after aspiration to rule out puncture of a blood vessel. The needle is then partially withdrawn and the remaining local anesthetic injected subcutaneously on each side of the anterior aspect of the root of the penis to block fibers arising from the ilioinguinal and genitofemoral nerves.

For this block the local anesthetic solution should be free of adrenaline. For children a dose of 0.2 ml/kg body weight is used; for adults a dose of less than 10 ml is sufficient.

Suggested reading

Soliman MG, Tremblay NA (1978) Nerve block of the penis for postoperative pain relief in children. Anesth Analg 57:495

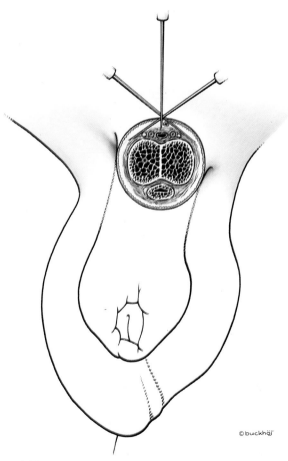

Fig. 2.59. Penile block. Anatomy and technique.

Fig. 2.60. Penile block. Circumferential subcutaneous infiltration after injection under Buck's fascia.

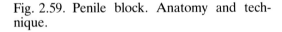
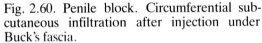
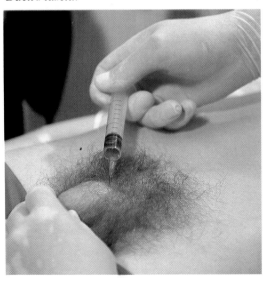

Paracervical block

For this block the patient is best positioned in the lithotomy position. After preparation of the vagina and vulva with a bactericidal solution the lateral fornices of the vagina are injected with local anesthetic solution.

A 12- to 14-cm 20 gauge needle with a guide is used. The guide serves to direct the needle properly and also to avoid insertion of the needle deeper than 1.5 cm into the uterosacral ligament, thereby minimizing the risk of intravascular injection.

Directed by the index and middle fingers. the guide is introduced in the lateral fornix of the vagina in the 3 o'clock position. The needle is introduced through the guide until contact is made with the mucosa. The needle is then advanced through the uterosacral ligament for a maximum distance of 1.5 cm. After careful aspiration to rule out an intravascular position, 10 – 15 ml of a local anesthetic solution is injected. The procedure is repeated on the other side in the 9 o'clock position.

For nonobstetric indications a 1% solution of a short-acting local anesthetic containing adrenaline or 0.25% bupivacaine with adrenaline can be used.
Toxic reactions have been reported so full resuscitative facilities should be available.

Suggested reading

Grimes DA, Cates W Jr (1976) Deaths from paracervical anesthesia used for first-trimester abortion. N Engl J Med 295:1397

Svancarek W, Chirino O, Schaefer G Jr et al. (1977) Retropsoas and subgluteal abscesses following paracervical and pudendal anesthesia. JAMA 237:892

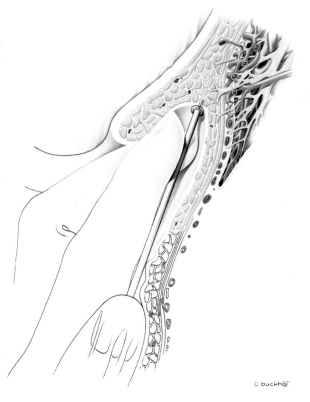

Fig. 2.61. Paracervical block. Technique of injection in the lateral formix. Note the guide that prevents too deep an insertion of the needle.

© buckhöj

3. Surgical indications

Introduction

All surgery of the body can be carried out under nerve block or infiltration analgesia. One need only to refer to the monumental works of pioneers such as Braun, Farr, Labat and Pitkin to note the scope of regional analgesia as it was used during the first decades of this century. The exquisite details of anatomy, the meticulous anatomic dissections, and the expansive clinical experience that these physicians obtained cannot easily be accomplished in the current medical environment.

The major motivating force, of course, was the necessity to provide operating conditions satisfactory for the proposed surgery. An overriding fear prevalent at the time was the high morbidity and mortality rate associated with the use of general anesthesia. These feelings are exemplified by a statement from Pitkin's classic **Conduction Anesthesia:** *"The author, having been perturbed by the unhappy postoperative state of patients who had taken drop ether for this and other operative procedures early began to cast about for better methods, and for more than 20 years now has done every radical mastectomy under nerve block anesthesia."* The anesthesia required superficial cervical plexus block, brachial plexus block, and intercostal block of the second to ninth intercostal nerves. Similar techniques are described for almost all surgical procedures where combinations of somatic and autonomic blocks were used for operations on thoracic and abdominal viscera. As late as 1948 most cholecystectomies in Uppsala were performed under "Kappi's block," i.e., a combination of hypobaric spinal analgesia and splanchnic nerve block. In a series of papers published between 1928 and 1942 the New York surgeon Harry Koster described the use of a standardized total spinal analgesia for a wide variety of surgical procedures, including mastoidectomies, craniotomies and nose repairs. The patient material comprised almost 20 000, ranging from newborn babies to nonagenarians. The anesthesia-related morbidity and mortality were very low even when compared with the figures of today.

Anesthesiology has progressed immensely over the last few decades and the technically more demanding, and probably in most hands less effective, nerve blocking techniques were replaced by modern inhalation or intravenous anesthesia in the 1950s. Only in specific institutions or areas, such as Scandinavia, has regional analgesia enjoyed significant popularity.

In recent years a renewed interest in these techniques has emerged as investigations have shown that regional analgesia has definite merits when compared with general anesthesia in terms of various metabolic, circulatory, ventilatory and hormonal responses to surgically inflicted trauma. When dealing with elderly and more debilitated patients it has become evident that there is another major advantage of regional analgesia, namely the ability to sustain it into the postoperative period providing for a more benign surgical recovery.

Suggested reading

Aitkenhead AR, Wishart HY, Pebbles Brown DA (1978) High spinal nerve block for large bowel anastomosis. A retrospective study. Br J Anaesth 50:117

Bergman H (1970) Die derzeitige Stellung der Lokalanaesthesie. In: Hutschenreuter K, Bihler K, Fritsche P (eds) Anaesthesie in extremen Altersklassen. (Anaesthesiology and resuscitation, vol 47) Springer, Berlin, p 219

Bonica JJ (1984) History, current status and future of regional anesthesia. Ann Chir Gynaecol 73:108

Brandt MR, Fernandes A, Mordhorst R et al. (1978) Epidural analgesia improves postoperative nitrogen balance. Br Med J I:1106

Bredbacka S, Blombäck M, Hägnevik K et al (1986) Per- and postoperative changes in coagulation and fibrinolytic variables during abdominal hysterectomy under epidural or general anaesthesia. Acta Anaesthesiol Scand 30:204

Buckley FPP, Robinson B, Simonowitz DA et al. (1983) Anaesthesia in the morbidly obese. A comparison of anaesthetic and analgesic requirements for upper abdominal surgery. Anaesthesia 38:840

Chin SP, Abou-Madi MN, Eurin B et al. (1982) Blood loss in total hip replacement; extradural versus phenoperidine analgesia. Br J Anaesth 54:491

Cooper GM, Holdcroft A, Hall GM et al. (1979) Epidural analgesia and the metabolic response to surgery. Can Anaesth Soc J 26:381

Davis FM, Laurenson VG (1981) Spinal anaesthesia or general anaesthesia for emergency hip surgery in elderly patients. Anaesth Intensive Care 9:352

Enquist A, Brandt MR, Fernandes A et al. (1977) The blocking effects of epidural analgesia on the adrenocortical and hyperglycemic response to surgery. Acta Anaesthesiol Scand 21:330

Enquist A, Fog-Möller F, Christiansen C et al. (1980) Influence of epidural analgesia on the catecholamine and cyclic AMP responses to surgery. Acta Anaesthesiol Scand 24:17

Farr RE (1929) Practical local anesthesia and its surgical technic, 2nd edn. Henry Kimpton, London, p 431

Flatt JR, Birrell PC, Hobbes A (1984) Effects of anaesthesia on some aspects of mental functioning of surgical patients. Anaesth Intens Care 12:315

Håkansson E, Rutberg H, Jorfeldt L et al. (1985) Effects of the extradural administration of morphine or bupivacaine on the metabolic response to upper abdominal surgery. Br J Anaesthesiol 57:394

Hendolin H, Mattila MAK, Poikolainen E (1981) The effect of lumbar epidural analgesia on the development of deep vein thrombosis of the legs after open prostatectomy. Acta Chir Scand 147:425

Hjortsö N-C, Christensen NJ, Andersen T et al. (1985) Effects of the extradural administration of local anaesthetic agents and morphine on the urinary excretion of cortisol, catecholamines and nitrogen following abdominal surgery. Br J Anaesth 57:400

Hole A, Unsgaard G (1983) The effect of epidural and general anaesthesia on lymphocyte functions during and after major orthopedic surgery. Acta Anaesthesiol Scand 27:135

Hole A, Terjesen T, Breivik H (1980) Epidural versus general anaesthesia for total hip arthroplasty in elderly patients. Acta Anaesthesiol Scand 24:279

Hole A, Unsgaard G, Breivik H (1982) Monocyte functions are depressed during and after surgery under general anaesthesia but not under epidural anaesthesia. Acta Anaesthesiol Scand 26:301

Holmdahl M H:son (1981) Changing role of general versus regional anesthesia in clinical practice. In: Wüst HJ, Zindler M (eds) Neue Aspekte in der Regionalanaesthesie. (Anaesthesiology and intensive care medicine, vol 158). Springer, Berlin, p 143

Jörgensen BC, Andersen HB, Engquist A (1982) Influence of epidural morphine on postoperative pain, endocrine-metabolic, and renal responses to surgery. A controlled study. Acta Anaesthesiol Scand 26:63

Karhunen U, Jönn G (1982) A comparison of memory function following local and general anaesthesia for extraction of senile cataract. Acta Anaesthesiol Scand 26:291

Katz J (1973) A survey of anesthetic choice among anesthesiologists. Anesth Analg 52:373

Kehlet H (1978) Influence of epidural analgesia on the endocrine-metabolic response to surgery. Acta Anaesthesiol Scand (Suppl) 70:39

Kehlet H (1982) The modifying effect of general and regional anaesthesia on the endocrine – metabolic response to surgery. Reg Anaesth 7:S38

Kehlet H (1984) Should regional anesthesia and pharmacological agents such as beta blockers and opiates be utilized in modulating pain response? J Trauma 24:S177

Kehlet H (1984) Epidural analgesia and the endocrine-metabolic response to surgery. Update and perspectives. Acta Anaesthesiol Scand 28:125

Kehlet H (1984) Does regional anaesthesia reduce post-operative morbidity? Intensive Care Med 10:165

Kehlet H (1984) Influence of regional anaesthesia on postoperative morbidity. Ann Chir Gynaecol 73:171

Kehlet H, Brandt MR, Prange-Hanson A et al. (1979) Effect of epidural analgesia on metabolic profiles during and after surgery. Br J Surg 66:543

Keith J (1977) Anaesthesia and blood loss in total hip replacement. Anaesthesia 32:444

Koster H (1928) Spinal anesthesia. With special reference to its use in surgery of the head, neck and thorax. Am J Surg V(6):554

Koster H, Wolf N (1930) Spinal anesthesia in mastoid surgery. Arch Otolaryngol 12:591

Labat G (1923) Regional anesthesia. Its technic and clinical application. WB Saunders, Philadelphia.

McKenzie PJ, Wishart HY, Dewar KMS et al. (1980) Comparison of the effects of spinal anaesthesia and general anaesthesia on postoperative oxygenation and perioperative mortality. Br J Anaesth 52:49

McKenzie PJ, Wishart HY, Smith G (1984) Longterm outcome after repair of fractured neck of femur. Comparison of subarachnoid and general anaesthesia. Br J Anaesth 56:581

McLaren AD, Stockwell MC, Reid VT (1978) Anaesthetic techniques for surgical correction of fractured neck of femur. Anaesthesia 33:10

Modig J (1976) Respiration and circulation after total hip replacement surgery. A comparison between parenteral analgesics and continuous lumbar epidural block. Acta Anaesthesiol Scand 20:225

Modig J (1978) Lumbar epidural nerve blockade versus parenteral analgesics. Acta Anaesthesiol Scand (Suppl) 70:30

Modig J, Malmberg P, Karlström G (1980) Effect of epidural versus general anaesthesia on calf blood flow. Acta Anaesthesiol Scand 24:305

Modig J, Hjelmstedt Ä, Sahlstedt B et al. (1981) Comparative influences of epidural and general anaesthesia on deep venous thrombosis and pulmonary embolism after total hip replacement. Acta Chir Scand 147:125

Modig J, Borg T, Bagge L et al. (1983) Role of extradural and of general anaesthesia in fibrinolysis and coagulation after total hip replacement. Br J Anaesth 55:625

Modig J, Borg T, Karlström G et al. (1983) Thromboembolism after total hip replacement: role of epidural and general anaesthesia. Anesth Analg 62:174

Möller IW, Rem J, Brandt MR et al. (1982) Effect of posttraumatic epidural analgesia on the cortisol and hyperglycemic response to surgery. Acta Anaesthesiol Scand 6:56

Möller IW, Hjortsö N-C, Krantz T et al. (1984) The modifying effect of spinal anaesthesia on intra- and postoperative adrenocortical and hyperglycaemic response to surgery. Acta Anaesthesiol Scand 28:266

Murphy TM (1984) When is regional the anesthetic technique of choice? American Society of Anesthesiologists Annual Refresher Course Lectures. 107:1

Nimmo WS, Littlewood DG, Scott DB et al. (1978) Gastric emptying following hysterectomy with extradural analgesia. Br J Anaesth 50:559

Pflug AE, Halter JB (1981) Effect of spinal anesthesia on adrenergic tone and the neuro-endocrine response to surgical stress in humans. Anesthesiology 55:120

Pitkin GP (1946) Conduction anesthesia. Lippincott/Harper & Row, New York

Rem J, Brandt MR, Kehlet H (1980) Prevention of postoperative lymphopenia and granulocytosis by epidural analgesia. Lancet I:283

Renck H (1969) The elderly patient after anaesthesia and surgery. Acta Anaesthesiol Scand (Suppl) 34

Renck H (1983) The proportion of regional anesthesia for surgery in Sweden, Norway, and Finland. Reg Anesth 8:144

Riis J, Lomholt B, Haxholdt O et al. (1983) Immediate and long-term mental recovery from general versus epidural anaesthesia in elderly patients. Acta Anaesthesiol Scand 27:44

Rosberg B, Fredin H, Gustafson C (1982) Anaesthetic techniques and surgical blood loss in total hip arthroplasty. Acta Anaesthesiol Scand 26:189

Schonwald G, Fish KJ, Perkash I (1981) Cardiovascular complications during anesthesia in spinal cord injured patients. Anesthesiology 55:550

Stefansson T, Wikström T, Haljamäe H (1982) Effects of neurolept and epidural analgesia on cardiovascular function and tissue metabolism in the geriatric patient. Acta Anaesthesiol Scand 26:386

Stjernström H, Henneberg S, Eklund A et al.(1985) Thermal balance during transurethral resection of the prostate. A comparison of general anaesthesia and epidural analgesia. Acta Anaesthesiol Scand 29:743

Thorburn J, London JR, Vallance R (1980) Spinal and general anaesthesia in total hip replacement: frequency of deep vein thrombosis. Br J Anaesth 52:1117

Whelan P, Morris PJ (1982) Immunological responsiveness after transurethral resection of the prostate: General versus spinal anaesthetic. Clin Exp Immunol 48:611

General/Regional

Johnson A, Bengtsson M, Merits H et al (1986) Anesthesia for major hip surgery. A clinical study of spinal and general anesthesia in 244 patients. Reg Anesth 11:83

Modig J, Maripuu E, Sahlstedt B (1986) Thromboembolism following total hip replacement. A prospective investigation of 94 patients with emphasis on the efficacy of lumbar epidural anesthesia in prophylaxis. Reg Anesth 11:72

Regional block for surgical procedures of the chest wall

The use of intercostal nerve blocks for a variety of surgical procedures of the chest wall is relatively simple to accomplish with minimal to no systemic effects to the patient. Procedures such as rib resection, thoracocentesis, scar revision, mammoplasy, and mastectomy can all be performed with the use of multiple intercostal or paravertebral blocks.

For procedures on the anterior chest wall intercostal blocks performed behind the posterior axillary line will usually suffice. It must be remembered that because of the overlapping innervation of the intercostal nerves a minimum of three blocks is required for any surgical intervention. As a general rule the segmental nerve to the dermatomes cephalad and caudad to the incision should always be blocked. For procedures closer to the midline of the back, such as repairs of soft tissue or bony injury, paravertebral blocks are indicated. When the procedure is to be done bilaterally and is somewhat extensive a thoracic epidural might be the block of choice.

A straightforward technique for the performance of a simple mastectomy under regional anesthesia has been described on p 135.

Regional blocks for surgical procedures of the upper abdominal wall

For procedures such as cholecystostomy, gastrostomy, repair of incisional hernia, and drainage of abscesses, blocks of the sixth through tenth intercostal nerves will provide a field of analgesia from the xiphoid process to the level of the umbilicus. These need only be carried out unilaterally for procedures such as cholecystostomy but must be bilateral for procedures in which the incision will come near to or cross the midline. The blocks should be done behind the posterior axillary line in either case. This will provide not only skin analgesia but also muscle relaxation since these nerves are the motor supply to the abdominal wall musculature. In addition the parietal peritoneum will be anesthetized.

Regional blocks for thoracotomies

Although there are anecdotal reports on thoracotomies performed under thoracic epidural analgesia alone, this technique could not be recommended today. Thoracic epidural analgesia in combination with a light general anesthesia and positive pressure ventilation offers a very stable intraoperative anesthetic as well as the potential for providing postoperative pain relief.

For a lateral thoracotomy for a lung operation, a continuous epidural through a puncture at the T3 – T4 interspace is recommended since punctures at the T5 – T8 levels are usually more difficult to accomplish due to the narrow vertebral interspaces. The catheter should be secured in such a position that it will not interfere with the preparation and dressing of the area of skin incision. For intraoperative analgesia we use an initial dose of 6 – 8 ml of an appropriate local anesthetic. Top up doses intraoperatively of 3 – 4 ml are given at 1- to 2-hourly intervals, depending on the drug used. For concomitant light general anesthesia nitrous oxide-oxygen with minimal amounts of narcotics and/or barbiturates is all that is required. The patient should be kept slightly hyperventilated. When the parietal pleura is opened, FiO_2 should be increased to 0.4 – 0.5.

We have also performed a series of thymectomies, for the treatment of myasthenia gravis, via a median sternotomy employing this technique. It was possible to obtain excellent operating conditions, as well as postoperative analgesia, with minimal amounts of drugs, avoiding medications such as neuromuscular blocking agents and opioids which perhaps could have worsened the underlying disease and necessitated prolonged artificial ventilation postoperatively.

It has been shown that a median sternotomy, performed for aortocoronary bypass grafting, even in heavily narcotized patients, causes untoward circulatory effects that jeopardize the myocardial oxygen supply. It might seem surprising that regional anesthetic techniques have not been used regularly in order to effectively block the nociceptive input from this part of the procedure.

Because of the risk of intraspinal hemorrhage during heparinization, an epidural technique might be considered inadvisable. On the other hand it seems logical to use either bilateral blocks of the first through sixth intercostal nerves or the technically less demanding field block of the sternum. For the latter technique skin wheals are raised on both sides of the sternum over the rib cartilages. A 5-cm 22 gauge needle is inserted perpendicularly and advanced to the cartilage. It is then inclined cephalad and gently advanced 0.5 cm deeper to the external surface of the cartilage and 3 ml of 0.5% bupivacaine is injected fanwise. The needle is then partially withdrawn and redirected caudad over the cartilage and the space below is injected similarly. The other spaces are injected similarly and the procedure is completed by joining the wheals by subcutaneous infiltration of 0.125% – 0.25% bupivacaine.

Suggested reading

Bromage PR (1978) Epidural analgesia. WB Saunders, Philadelphia, p 486

Crawford OB, Ottosen P, Buckingham WW et al. (1951) Peridural anesthesia in thoracic surgery, a review of 677 cases. Anesthesiology 12:73

Labat G (1923) Regional anesthesia. Its technic and clinical application. WB Saunders, Philadelphia, p 333

Vasconcelos E (1944) Cancer of the esophagus: original technique for total esophagectomy. Dis Chest X:471

Regional blocks for intra-abdominal procedures

For these procedures analgesia not only of the abdominal wall but also of the abdominal content is necessary to interrupt sensory and autonomic reflexes secondary to manipulation or traction. A laparotomy performed under regional anesthesia alone requires the hands of a gentle and skilled surgeon.

Somatic nerve block is preferably achieved by thoracic epidural anesthesia instituted at a level corresponding to the midpoint of the dermatomal level of the incision. The block should encompass the origin of the splanchnic nerves, i.e., extend to the T5 level, in order to produce a sympathetic denervation of the splanchnic area. As an alternative multiple intercostal nerve blocks could also be used but these do not include the sympathetic efferents to the splanchnic nerves.

For high laparotomies it is necessary also to block the vagal innervation of the splanchnic area. In the past surgeons performed a celiac plexus block by the infiltration of a local anesthetic around the celiac artery once the abdomen was opened under regional anesthesia. Presently surgeons lack this experience and prefer the anesthesiologist to perform the block via a posterior approach (see p 157).

In order to avoid inflicting unnecessary pain, one should perform the epidural block, wait 2–4 min for its initial onset, and then proceed with the celiac plexus block with the patient still in the lateral position. For long-lasting operations a continuous technique employing a catheter could be used. In experienced hands the combined procedure as described here will only take around 15–20 min and cause little discomfort to the patient. The technique is very useful for selected patients, i.e., those who absolutely refuse general anesthesia. During the combined blockade, employing continuous techniques, it is possible to perform even major intra-abdominal surgery such as aortoiliac bypass procedures. It is gratifying to note that high-risk patients frequently request their glasses, a newspaper and food within a couple of hours after such procedures.

Another advantage of regional anesthesia, alone or in combination with very light general anesthesia (nitrous oxide-oxygen) intraoperatively or for postoperative pain relief, is that the risk of disruption of bowel anastomoses and its associated mortality seems to be reduced. The reasons might be increased blood flow to the bowel and reduced tension at the anastomosis site due to avoidance of neostigmine and narcotic analgesics.

In order to reduce incisional and postoperative pain less extensive regional techniques such as various abdominal field blocks might be used. The operation requires concomitant general anesthesia which, however, could be kept lighter than when no field block is used.

For upper abdominal midline or pararectal incisions the following technique can be used: With the patient in the supine position skin wheals are raised along the costal margins and the lateral margins of the recti muscles. One is made at the tip of the xiphoid process, one on each side at the lateral margin of the insertion of the rectus muscle at the costal margin and one on each side on the lateral margin of the rectus muscle slightly cephalad of the umbilicus. For injection through the lateral wheals a 8- to 10-cm 22 gauge needle is used. After piercing the skin the needle is gently advanced in the superficial abdominal fascia toward the rectus muscle. As soon as the needle touches the rectus sheath, it is advanced 0.5 – 1 cm and about 2 ml of the local anesthetic is injected. The needle tip is then withdrawn subcutaneously and reintroduced more and more cephalad and then caudad, each time injecting a small amount of the local anesthetic within the rectus sheath. Injections into the rectus sheath and the rectus muscle are done through the other skin wheals using a total of up to 40 ml of 0.25% bupivacaine with adrenaline. Finally 0.125% – 0.25% bupivacaine with adrenaline is infiltrated subcutaneously along the lines joining all wheals.

Field block for low midline incisions is administered by distributing 0.25% bupivacaine with adrenaline within the rectus sheath along the lateral margin of the recti muscles from the pubes to a little above the umbilicus as described above. From the most caudad point of injection the local anesthetic is also injected in close contact with the pubis and behind it in the prevesical space. This injection should be made after repeated aspirations as this area is very rich in thin-walled veins.

Provided the injections in the rectal sheath are performed laterally, before the segmental nerves give off their branches to the rectal muscles and the peritoneum, the block is accompanied by relaxation of the rectal muscles and analgesia of the parietal peritoneum.

Suggested reading

Aitkenhead AR (1984) Anesthesia for bowel surgery. Ann Chir Gynaecol 73:177

Bigler D, Hjortsö N-C, Kehlet H (1985) Disruption of colonic anastomosis during continuous epidural analgesia. Anaesthesia 40:278

Farr RE (1929) Practical local anesthesia and its surgical technic, 2nd edn. Henry Kimpton, London, p 431

Kappis M (1919) Sensibilität und lokale Anästhesie im chirurgischen Gebiet der Bauchhöle mit besonderer Berücksichtigung der Splanchnicus-Anästhesie, Bruns' Beiträge zur klin Chirurgie. 115:161

Labat G (1923) Regional anesthesia. Its technic and clinical application. W.B. Saunders, Philadelphia, p 348

Quimby CW (1972) Intercostal-celiac plexus block for abdominal surgery in the poor risk patient. J Arkansas Med Soc 68:266

Satoyoshi M, Kamiyama Y (1980) Caudal Anaesthesia for upper abdominal surgery in infants and children: a simple calculation of volume of local anaesthetic. Acta Anaesthesiol Scand 28:57

Treissmann DA (1980) Disruption of colonic anastomosis associated with epidural anesthesia. Reg Anesth 5:22

Tsuji H, Shirasaka C, Asoh T et al.(1983) Influence of splanchnic nerve blockade on endocrine-metabolic responses to upper abdominal surgery. Br J Surg 70:437

Comparison of techniques

Laparotomies can only be performed under epidural – preferably segmental – or multiple intercostal blocks combined with a splanchnic or celiac block. In order to be able to reduce the depth of general anesthesia and to provide good postoperative analgesia, an abdominal field block is a very reasonable alternative. It must be considered a simple and safe procedure which is not associated with risks of circulatory and/or respiratory complications.

Older textbooks in regional anesthesia devote considerable space to the various abdominal field blocks but to our knowledge they are rarely applied today. The more technically demanding epidural and intercostal blocks might better satisfy the professional pride of today's anesthesiologists. Considering the simplicity and safety of field blocks and the fact that they can be used in subsequently heparinized patients we think that these blocks deserve more widespread use than is presently the case.

Combined regional and general anesthesia

Often it is advantageous to combine the use of a regional blocking technique with a light state of general anesthesia.

Surgical anesthesia includes hypnosis, analgesia, muscle relaxation, and suppression of various reflexes. While in the past diethyl ether by inhalation accomplished all these effects, today balanced anesthesia is used. This implies a combination of agents, each inducing one or several of the above objectives. Regional nerve block results in a temporary, complete interruption of transmission in autonomic, sensory and motor nerves and thereby fulfills three of the four mentioned components. To accomplish the fourth, hypnosis, only light general anesthesia has to be added.

General anesthesia with inhalation and/or intravenous agents can produce an analgesic state equivalent to that of regional anesthesia only when high dosages are employed. These dosages have depressant effects on all major organ systems in the body and considerably prolong the recovery period. Still, they do not completely eliminate the various reflex effects of surgical stimulation.

In patients with limited cardiorespiratory reserves or significant hypertension the extensive analgesic component that is provided by regional analgesia will make the intra- and postoperative course much smoother than when various combinations of inhalational and intravenous agents are used. There are generally few alarming incidents when "balanced anesthesia" is accomplished by a combination of thoracic epidural block, 70% N_2O in O_2, and controlled ventilation.

We suggest doing the block prior to induction of general anesthesia. This has the advantage of permitting the anesthesiologist to verify the onset and distribution of the block and to avoid neurological complications secondary to it, i.e., neural puncture or intraneural injections. In addition it may abate the untoward circulatory effects of endotracheal intubation.

Field block for inguinal hernia repair

This procedure has been described on p 145 As a rule it requires that the surgeon supplement the initial block during the progress of surgery.

Hernia repair under local anesthesia has two definite merits, both reducing the frequency of recurrences. Firstly, any indirect hernia can be visualized by asking the patient to cough intraoperatively. Secondly, the same technique can be used at the end of operation to test the adequacy of the repair. Occasionally a weakness can be identified and corrected.

In children regional anesthesia in the form of a combined ilioinguinal and iliohypogastric nerve block can be used, after induction of general anesthesia, employing 0.5 ml/year of 0.5% bupivacaine without adrenaline. This technique significantly reduces early postoperative pain, which is considered particularly useful in pediatric day-stay surgery.

Suggested reading

Flanagan LJr, Bascom JU (1984) Repair of groin hernia. Outpatient approach with local anesthesia. Surg Clin North Am 64:257

Glassow F (1984) Inguinal hernia repair using local anesthesia. Ann R Coll Surg Engl 66:382

Hannallah RS, Broadman LM, Belman AB et al (1984) Control of postorchidopexy pain in paediatric outpatients: comparision of two regional techniques. Anesthesiology 61:A429

Shandling B, Steward DJ (1980) Regional analgesia for postoperative pain in paediatric outpatient surgery. J Paediatr Surg 15:477

Smith BAC, Jones SEF (1982) Analgesia after herniotomy in a paediatric day unit. Br Med J 285:1466

Nerve blocks for urologic procedures

Kidney operations through a lateral incision

The pain from this incision can easily be handled by many different block procedures. In our experience blocks of the eleventh and twelfth intercostal nerves do not suffice but should be supplemented by paravertebral blocks of the first and second lumbar nerves. These blocks can very easily be performed when the patient is positioned on the operating table. The techniques of the blocks have been described on p 140. It should be reemphaized that despite apparent correct placement of the needles for paravertebral block a subarachnoid puncture can result. Therefore the position of the needle must always be checked as carefully as possible before injection.

A total dose of less than 20 ml of 0.5% bupivacaine with adrenaline is sufficient.

Suggested reading

Crawford ED, Skinner DG (1982) Intercostal nerve block with thoracoabdominal and flank incisions. Urology 19:25

Humphreys CF, Kay H (1976) The control of postoperative wound pain with the use of bupivacaine injections. J Urol 116:618

Noller CW, Gillenwater JY, Howards SS et al. (1977) Intercostal nerve blocks with flank incision. J Urol 117:759

Bladder and prostate operations

Transurethral procedures are generally considered a major indication for spinal or epidural blocks as these provide the surgeon with the best operating conditions and cause less intra- and postoperative bleeding. Usually a segmental level to T10 is considered sufficient. When analgesia is restricted to that level intraoperative pain is considered to indicate a surgical perforation of the bladder. We must admit, however, that we usually employ a somewhat higher level for the analgesia to provide a complete relaxation of the abdominal wall, and so far we have not encountered any unrecognized cases of intraoperative bladder perforation.

The block must sometimes be supplemented by injection of the obturator nerve on one or both sides (see p 147). This is due to the fact that cautery of a bladder tumor located close to the site of the obturator nerve will cause uncontrollable adductions of the leg, thereby complicating the work of the surgeon and increasing the risk of bladder perforation.

In the choice between spinal and epidural anesthetics it should be kept in mind that the procedures can be long and postoperative pain relief may be indicated. In these cases continuous epidural anesthesia is preferred to the standard spinal block.

Suggested reading

Yazaki T, Ishikawa H, Kanoh S et al (1985) Accurate obturator nerve block in transurethral surgery. Urology 26:588

Meatotomy, circumcision

Meatotomy and circumcision can be performed on an outpatient basis employing either caudal blocks (p 122) or penile blocks (p 148). Penile block will provide a long-lasting postoperative analgesia without any motor block or interference with micturition.

In children these techniques, in combination with light general anesthesia, are very rewarding and easily done. For caudal anesthesia a dose of 0.5 ml/year gives a very predictable five segment block. In order to avoid voiding problems a short-acting agent might be preferable. For penile blocks solutions free of adrenaline should always be used.

Suggested reading

Bacon AK (1977) An alternative for post circumcision pain. Anaesth Intens Care 5:63

Blaise G, Roy WL (1984) Postoperative pain relief after hypospadias repair in pediatric patients: regional anesthesia vs systemic analgesics. Anesthesiology 61:A430

Holve RL, Bromberg PJ, Groveman HD et al. (1983) Regional anesthesia during newborn circumcision. Clin Pediatr 22:813

Jensen BH (1981) Caudal block for postoperative pain relief in children after genital operations. A comparison between bupivacaine and morphine. Acta Anaesthesiol Scand 25:373

Martin LVH (1982) Postoperative analgesia after circumcision in children. Br J Anaesth 54:1263

May AE, Wandless J, James RH (1982) Analgesia for circumcision in children. A comparison of caudal bupivacaine and intramuscular buprenorphine. Acta Anaesthesiol Scand 26:331

Sara CA, Lowry CJ (1984) A complication of circumcision and dorsal nerve block of the penis. Anaesth Intens Care 13:79

Vater M, Wandless J (1985) Caudal or dorsal nerve block? A comparison of two local anaesthetic techniques for postoperative analgesia following day case circumcision. Acta Anaesthesiol Scand 29:175

White, J, Harrison B, Rickmond P et al. (1983) Postoperative analgesia for circumcision. Br Med J 286:1934

Yeoman PM, Cooke R, Hain WR (1983) Penile block for circumcision? A comparison with caudal blockade. Anaesthesia 38:862

Cystoscopy

In males as well as females an adequately performed topical anesthesia is usually sufficient. For outpatients with bladderneck obstruction caudal analgesia is sometimes indicated. It must, however, be remembered that in adults caudal analgesia is sometimes difficult to perform and very often unpredictable.

Nerve blocks for gynecologic procedures

Dilatation and curettage

In most cases this procedure is performed under light intravenous or inhalational anesthesia. For patients refusing general anesthesia or with a full stomach a paracervical block will provide satisfactory operating conditions.

Conization

This procedure is most frequently performed under light general anesthesia However, in some institutions it is regularly performed under a combination of paracervical block and light intravenous anesthesia which offers quite adequate intraoperative and superior postoperative conditions.

Low laparotomies

Hysterectomies are not usually performed under regional or combined regional and general anesthesia. The reasons are not clear but obviously both anesthesiologists and surgeons must be satisfied with what general anesthesia provides. On the other hand these operations can be performed under spinal or epidural anesthesia quite readily.

Insertion of radioactive packs for irradiation therapy of gynecological cancers requires anesthesia for dilatation of the cervix, frequently for curettage, insertion of the probe, and packing. The use of paracervical block in combination with light general anesthesia significantly reduces recovery time and thereby the time for which recovery room personnel are exposed to irradiation.

Nerve blocks for proctologic procedures

Several factors speak in favor of regional instead of general anesthesia for these procedures. First of all they are usually performed in the prone position so a general endotracheal anesthetic has to be given for even a minor procedure; secondly they are not infrequently performed in elderly or debilitated patients; and thirdly they are often followed by postoperative sphincter spasms. Caudal or saddle block or low spinal anesthesia could be used. Caudal block has several advantages:

1. Minimal circulatory effects
2. Not effected by position
3. Useful for out patients

As mentioned before, this technique is occasionally unsuccessful. In hospitalized patients spinal anesthesia may therefore be of some advantage.

Nerve blocks for post-thoracotomy pain relief

Nerve blocks for post-thoracotomy pain relief are an important adjunct to other pharmacologic methods. They lack the central depressant effects of opioids and can be of great help in the mobilization of the patient as well as in ensuring patient cooperation during chest physiotherapy.

Intercostal nerve blocks, performed either at the time of surgery or in the postoperative period, have been shown to provide good, but not total analgesia in patients after thoracic surgical procedures. As usually performed, the dorsal ramus of the nerve and its midback innervation is not anesthetized. Thus the posterior part of the surgical incision lies outside of the anesthetized area. In addition, pain after thoracotomy also in part stems from visceral stimulation (from the pleura) as well as from muscle and ligament stretching and tearing caused by the opening of rib retractors.

When performed by the surgeon from the inside of the thoracic cavity the blocks can be performed proximally, thus including the posterior ramus. These proximal internal intercostal nerve blocks have resulted in total spinals, however.

Thoracic epidural block has several advantages and disadvantages when used for post-thoracotomy pain. The major advantage is that it provides both visceral and somatic analgesia which can be extended for several days when a continuous technique is used. The major disadvantage is that it causes an extensive sympathetic block with associated risk of circulatory complications. This effect is dose-dependent and rarely occurs when top-up doses of 4 ml or less are used. The amount of painrelief obtained is also dosedependent, so that the "therapeutic range," i.e., the difference between the dose needed for pain relief and the dose that causes hypotension, may sometimes be very narrow or even negative. Extreme care in the constant evaluation of dose requirements and the supervision of patients is strongly recommended in order to avoid circulatory complications.

Opioids could be used for post-thoracotomy pain relief by epidural administration. When morphine is employed it spreads very widely in the CSF, and lumbar administration might be feasible.

In some institutions thoracic epidural analgesia is induced postoperatively for pain relief following open heart surgery after heparin reversal. In addition to pain relief this technique reduces circulatory afterload and thereby cardiac work and acts as an antiarrhythmic.

Cryoanalgesia is a new technique which is being used for the management of post-thoracotomy pain. Briefly, cryoanalgesia is a method of freezing nerves so that they will no longer transmit neural impulses. This is done by the application of a cryoprobe directly on a peripheral nerve. A cryoprobe is a device which has a conducting metal tip in which a fine micropore opening exists through which a gas is forced under pressure. As the gas expands in the tip of the needle it cools very rapidly. When the metal tip comes into contact with any fluid-containing tissue, the fluid freezes, forming ice crystals. When nitrous oxide is used a temperature of −60°C results.

When the cryoprobe is placed in contact with an intercostal nerve and activated for a period of 1 min a cryolesion will be immediately generated. This lesion has several characteristics:

1. Endoneural edema proximally
2. Separation and disruption of myelinated fibers
3. Margination of white blood cells in some blood vessel walls
4. Extravasation of red blood cells into the endoneural space
5. No loss of nerve support structures – therefore nerve regrowth occurs in an orderly fashion

Physiologically, nerve function is interrupted. Nerve regeneration starts shortly after the frozen lesion has thawed. In about 1 month onset of recovery of the nerve can be noticed, with complete recovery taking from 3 to 6 months. Since the nerve regenerates within its own supporting matrix there will be no neuroma formation. In our experience with the technique there have been no untoward sequelae in terms of permanent nerve damage or neuritis. Wound healing proceeds normally.

The advantage of cryoanalgesia is that it produces a prolonged nerve block at one sitting. The major difficulty with cryoanalgesia is that the probe tip must lie directly on the nerve in order to be of maximum effectiveness. This is very easy to achieve when it is applied directly to the exposed intercostal nerve inside the chest at the time of surgery but is obviously more difficult when percutaneous route is employed.

Suggested reading

Arthur DS (1980) Postoperative thoracic epidural analgesia in children. Anaesthesia 35:1131

Benumof JL, Semenza J (1975) Total spinal anesthesia following intrathoracic intercostal nerve blocks. Anesthesiology 43:124

Bergh NP, Dottori O, Löf BA et al. (1966) Effect of intercostal block on lung function after thoracotomy. Acta Anaesthesiol Scand 24:85

Bonica JJ (1983) Current status of postoperative pain therapy. In: Yokota T, Dubner R (eds) Current topics in pain research and therapy. Proceedings of the international symposium on pain. Kyoto, December 12–13, 1982. Excerpta Medica, Amsterdam, p 169

Bryant LR, Trinkle JK, Wood RE (1971) A technique for intercostal nerve block after thoracotomy. Ann Thorac Surg 11:388

Conacher ID, Paes ML, Jacobson L et al. (1983) Epidural analgesia following thoracic surgery. Anaesthesia 38:546

de la Rocha AG, Chambers RRT (1984) Pain amelioration after thoracotomy: a prospective, randomized study. Ann Thorac Surg 37:239

Delilkan AE, Yong NK, Ong SC (1973) Post-operative local analgesia for thoracotomy with direct bupivacaine intercostal blocks. Anaesthesia 28:561

Ecoffey C, Attia J, Samii K (1985) Analgesia and side effects following epidural morphine in children. Anesthesiology 63:A470

Faust RJ, Nauss LA (1976) Post thoracotomy intercostal nerve block: comparison of its effects on pulmonary function with those of intramuscular meperidine. Anesth Analg 55:542

Fleming WH, Sarafian LB (1977) Kindness pays dividends: the medical benefits of intercostal nerve block following thoracotomy. J Thorac Cardiovasc Surg 74:273

Gallo JAJr, Lebowitz PW, Battit GE et al. (1983) Complications of intercostal nerve blocks performed under direct vision during thoracotomy: a report of two cases. J Thorac Cardiovasc Surg 86:628

Galway JE, Caves PK, Dundee JW (1974) Effect of intercostal nerve blockage during operation on lung function and the relief of pain following thoracotomy. Br J Anaesth 47:730

Griffiths DPG, Drummond AW, Cameron JD (1975) Postoperative extradural analgesia following thoracic surgery. A feasibility study. Br J Anaesth 47:48

Hennek K, Sydow F-W (1984) Die thoracale Periduralanaesthesie zur intra- und postoperativen Analgesie bei Lungenresektionen. Reg Anaesth 7:115

Kaplan JA, Miller ED, Gallagher EG (1975) Postoperative analgesia for thoracotomy patients. Anesth Analg 54:773

Katz J, Nelson W, Forest R et al. (1980) Cryoanalgesia for post-thoracotomy pain. Lancet I:512

Meignier M, Souron R, Le Neel JC (1983) Postoperative dorsal epidural analgesia in the child with respiratory disability. Anesthesiology 59:473

Moore DC (1975) Intercostal block for postoperative somatic pain following surgery of thorax and upper abdomen. Br J Anaesth 47:284

Naumann CP (1980) Influence of different methods for postoperative pain relief on pulmonary function after thoracic surgery. In: Wöst HJ, Zindler M (eds) Neue Aspekte in der Regionalanaesthesie. (Anaesthesiology and intensive care medicine, vol 161). Springer, Berlin

Nelson KM, Vincent RG, Bourke RJ et al. (1974) Intraoperative intercostal nerve freezing to prevent postthoracotomy pain. Ann Thorac Surg 18:280

Olivet RT, Nauss LA, Payne WS (1980) A technique for continuous intercostal nerve block analgesia following thoracotomy. J Thorac Cardiovasc Surg 80:308

Orr IA, Keenan DJM, Dundee JW (1981) Improved pain relief after thoracotomy: use of cryoprobe and morphine infusion. Br Med J 283:945

Reiz S (1984) Postoperative pain relief and regional techniques. Ann Chir Gynaecol 73:166

Restelli L, Movilia P, Bossi L et al. (1984) Management of pain after thoracotomy: a technique of multiple intercostal nerve blocks. Anesthesiology 61:353

Shulman M, Sandler AN, Bradley JW et al. (1984) Postthoracotomy pain and pulmonary function following epidural and systemic morphine. Anesthesiology 61:569

Shuman RL, Peters RM (1976) Epidural anesthesia following thoracotomy in patients with chronic obstructive airway disease. J Thorac Cardiovasc Surg 71:82

Toledo-Pereyra LH, DeMeester TR (1979) Postoperative randomized evaluation of intrathoracic intercostal nerve block with bupivacaine on postoperative ventilatory function. Ann Thorac Surg 27:203

Welchew EA, Thornton JA (1982) Continuous thoracic epidural fentanyl. A comparison of epidural fentanyl with intramuscular papaveretum for postoperative pain. Anaesthesia 37:309

Willdeck-Lund, G., Edström, H. (1975) Etidocaine in intercostal nerve block for pain relief after thoracotomy; a comparison with bupivacaine. Acta Anaesthesiol Scand (Suppl) 60:33

Woltering EA, Flye MW, Huntley S et al. (1980) Evaluation of bupivacaine nerve blocks in the modification of pain and pulmonary function changes after thoracotomy. Ann Thorac Surg 30:122

Nerve blocks for post-laparotomy pain relief

The use of intercostal blocks to provide pain relief after surgery of the upper abdomen is quite feasible, and the technique receives greatest clinical usage after gallbladder surgery. Block of the sixth to eleventh intercostal nerves at the costal angle will provide hours of analgesia. When a long-acting local anesthetic is used, 8 – 12 h of relief might occur.

Continuous epidural analgesia with either local anesthetics or narcotics is used quite frequently. It is a common practice to include an epidural block in the "balanced" anesthetic technique for major abdominal surgery, be it visceral or vascular, and then to prolong the epidural component of the technique into the postoperative period for pain relief.

When local anesthetics are used the epidural will ideally be a segmental block covering the incision and involved visceral innervation. The technique is described on p 111 and the dosage regimen on p 116. It is strongly recommended that the distribution of cutaneous analgesia be determined at regular intervals in order to provide adequate but not too extensive a zone of analgesia. When intermittent doses are used distribution of cutaneous analgesia is determined by pinprick immediately before and 10 min after administration. Vital signs are monitored 5 – 10 min after the top-up dose in addition to the prior predetermined intervals. Adjustments of doses and dose intervals are made accordingly.

Narcotics could also be administered epidurally for postoperative pain relief. In this technique a small amount of a narcotic drug, e.g., 2 – 6 mg of preservative-free morphine or its equivalent in 4 – 8 cc of saline, is used. Ordinarily a solution containing 1 mg/ml is used. With the narcotics a nerve block per se is not performed, rather receptor activity in the substantia gelatinosa of the dorsal horn gray matter is blocked.

Morphine is poorly lipid-soluble and will spread widely within the CSF; it is thus unnecessary to use a segmental epidural technique when morphine is used. From a practical point of view this property means that morphine, even after lumbar epidural administration, may affect the respiratory center in the medulla. Respiratory depression may be delayed as long as 12 – 20 h after the morphine injection and it may be accentuated when the patient is given parenteral narcotics for any reason. It is therefore mandatory that the patient is kept under close supervision for up to 20 h after administration of the last dose of epidural morphine. Should respiratory depression or arrest ensue, conventional resuscitative efforts are undertaken and the patient is given naloxone 0.2–0.4 mg i.v.

Many patients report generalized itching, and urinary retention occurs frequently.

Although the intraspinal narcotics relieve postoperative pain they do not affect other sensations. The patient will respond to pinprick or other noxious stimuli on the skin. There are supposedly minimal to no effects on the autonomic nervous system with this technique.

It should be obvious that the performance of any block procedure – with the exception of uncomplicated intercostal blocks – for pain relief in the postoperative period requires close observation of the patient by experienced personnel. Modifications of dosage regimens must be undertaken frequently in order to obtain maximum benefit from any technique. Whether or not this can be done in a general ward or should be restricted to a specific hospital unit depends on the local situation.

However desirable complete analgesia in the postoperative period may be from a humanitarian point of view, it must never jeopardize the safety of the patient. In selected cases complete analgesia is highly desirable. For these patients' safety they are often best nursed in an ICU environment.

Suggested reading

Ablondi MA, Ryan JF, O'Connell CT et al (1966) Continuous intercostal nerve blocks for postoperative pain relief. Anesth Analg 45:185

Addison NV, Brear FA, Budd K et al (1974) Epidural analgesia following cholecystectomy. Br J Surg 61:850

Benhamou D, Samii K, Noviant Y (1983) Effect of analgesia on respiratory muscle function after upper abdominal surgery. Acta Anaesthesiol Scand 27:22

Bilsback P, Rolly G, Tampubolon O (1985) Efficacy of the extradural administration of lofentanil, buprenorphine or saline in the management of postoperative pain. A double-blind study. Br J Anaesth 57:943

Bonica JJ (1983) Current status of postoperative pain therapy. In: Yokota T, Dubner R (eds) Current topics in pain research and therapy. Proceedings of the international symposium on pain. Kyoto, December 12–13, 1982. Excerpta Medica, Amsterdam, p 169

Bonnet F, Blery H, Zatan M et al. (1984) Effect of epidural morphine on post-operative pulmonary dysfunction. Acta Anaesthesiol Scand 28:147

Bromage PR (1982) Epidural narcotics for postoperative pain relief. Reg Anesth 7:140

Chrubasik J, Meynadier J, Scherpereel P et al. (1985) The effect of epidural somatostatin on postoperative pain. Anesth Analg 64:1085

Cullen ML, Staren ED, El-Ganzouri A et al (1985) Continuous epidural infusion for analgesia after major abdominal operations: A randomized, prospective, double-blind study. Surgery 98:718

Engberg G (1985) Respiratory performance after upper abdominal surgery. A comparison of pain relief with intercostal blocks and centrally acting analgesics. Acta Anaesthesiol Scand 29:427

Finer B (1970) Studies on the variability in expiratory efforts before and after cholecystectomy. Br J Anaesth 54:479

Gustafsson LL, Schildt B, Jacobsen K (1982) Adverse effects of extradural and intrathecal opiates: report of a nationwide survey in Sweden. Br J Anaesth 54:479

Hjortsö N-C, Neumann P, Frosig F et al. (1985) A controlled study on the effect of epidural analgesia with local anaesthetics and morphine on morbidity after abdominal surgery. Acta Anaesthesiol Scand 29:790

Hojklaer Larsen V, Iversen AD, Christensen P et al. (1985) Post-operative pain treatment after upper abdominal surgery with epidural morphine at thoracic or lumbar level. Acta Anaesthesiol Scand 29:566

Hollmén A, Saukkonen J (1969) Zur postoperativen Schmerzausschaltung nach Oberbauchoperationen. Narkotica, Intercostalblockade und Epiduralanaesthesie und deren Einfluss auf die Atmung. Der Anaesthesist 18:298

Holmdahl M H:son, Sjögren S, Ström G et al. (1972) Clinical aspects of continuous epidural blockade for postoperative pain relief. Uppsala J Med Sci 77:47

Hustad S, Djurhuus JC, Husegaard HC et al. (1985) Effect of post-operative extradural morphine on lower urinary tract function. Acta Anaesthesiol Scand 29:183

Jones SEF, Beasley JM, Macfarlane WR et al (1984) Intrathecal morphine for postoperative pain relief in children. Br J Anaesth 56:137

Jensen PJ, Siem-Jörgensen P, Nielsen T et al. (1982) Epidural morphine by the sacral route for postoperative pain relief. Acta Anaesthesiol Scand 26:511

Martin R, Salbaing I, Blaise G et al. (1982) Epidural morphine for postoperative pain relief. A dose-response curve. Anesthesiology 56:423

Massey-Dawkins CJ (1975) The relief of postoperative pain with special reference to epidural block. Proc Roy Soc Med 68:409

Naguib M, Adu-Gyamfi Y, Absood GH et al. (1986) Epidural ketamine for postoperative analgesia. Can Anaesth Soc J 33:16

Pflug AE, Murphy TM, Butler SH et al (1974) The effects of postoperative peridural analgesia on pulmonary therapy and pulmonary complications. Anesthesiology 41:8

Rawal N, Sjöstrand UH, Dahlström B et al. (1982) Epidural morphine for postoperative pain relief: a comparative study with intramuscular narcotic and intercostal nerve block. Anesth Analg 61:93

Renck H (1978) Thoracic epidural analgesia in the relief of postoperative pain. Acta Anaesthesiol Scand (Suppl) 70:43

Reiz S (1984) Postoperative pain relief and regional techniques. Ann Chir Gynaecol 73:166

Rybro L, Schurizek BA, Petersen TK et al. (1982) Postoperative analgesia and lung function: a comparison of intramuscular with epidural morphine. Acta Anaesthesiol Scand 26:514

Scheinin B, Rosenberg PH (1982) Effect of prophylactic epidural morphine or bupivacaine on postoperative pain after upper abdominal surgery. Acta Anaesthesiol Scand 26:474

Scott DB, Schweitzer S, Thorn J (1982) Epidural block in postoperative pain relief. Reg Anesth 7:135

Spence AA, Smith G (1971) Postoperative analgesia and lung function: a comparison of morphine with extradural block. Br J Anaesth 43:144

Stenseth R, Sellevold O, Breivik H (1985) Epidural morphine for postoperative pain: experience in 1085 patients. Acta Anaesthesiol Scand 29:148

Weddel SJ, Ritter RR (1981) Serum levels following epidural administration of morphine and correlation with relief of postsurgical pain. Anesthesiology 54:210

4. Nonsurgical applications

Introduction

Before discussing individual procedures for a variety of painful conditions of the chest and abdomen it is necessary to understand the following.

Pain is a complex psychological – physiologic event. It can emanate from a myriad of disease processes as well as an infinite number of nonorganic etiologies; all pain arising from the latter will be termed "psychogenic".

Before performing any diagnostic or therapeutic nerve block procedure the etiology of the underlying pain must be understood and the pathophysiologic processes leading to the discomfort recognized. The fundamental remedy for any painful disorder is appropriate treatment of the underlying pathologic process. Nerve blocks are used as an aid in diagnosis, as an addition to the therapeutic regime, or as a tool in and of themselves to eliminate pain because other modalities either have failed or have unacceptably high morbidity or mortality associated with them.

The experienced practitioner of nerve block therapy fully realizes the limited scope and difficulties in interpretation of the results of their use. He knows not to get overenthusiastic about the results of any single block or short series of blocks in a particular patient and he is also very well aware of the effects of any invasive procedure, i.e., nerve blocks, on the psychological makeup of patients and their desire for relief at any price. Evaluation of the procedures which he undertakes must be as objective as possible, since preliminary investigations with nerve blocks will often lead to further therapies which put the patient at risk, e.g. neurosurgery, neurolytic blocks. It must be reemphazised that neurolytic blocks are undertaken only for painful conditions with proven etiologies.

From the above it follows that it is the responsibility of the involved anesthesiologist to understand fully the patient's pain condition, to evaluate the indications for a nerve block, to perform the block correctly, and not least to evaluate the results. It is advisable to require a complete medical workup of the patient by the referring physician and also to consult a more experienced colleague in doubtful cases. The patient must be fully informed about the pros and cons of the procedure and give an informed consent to the block.

Suggested reading

Bonica JJ (1958) Diagnostic and therapeutic blocks. A reappraisal based on 15 years experience. Anesth Analg 37:58

Bonica JJ (1974) Current role of nerve blocks in diagnosis and therapy of pain Adv Neurol 4:445

International Association for the Study of Pain: Subcommittee on Taxonomy (1986) Classification of chronic pain. Description of chronic pain syndromes and definitions of pain terms. Pain Suppl 3

Menges LJ (1981) Chronic pain patients: some psychological aspects. In: Lipton S (ed) Persistent pain: modern methods of treatment, vol 3. Academic Press, London, p 87

Nerve blocks for differential diagnosis of visceral, somatic, and/or psychogenic pain

The patient who presents with thoraco-abdominal pain of questionable etiology is often a diagnostic challenge. There are several approaches that may be taken from a nerve block point of view.

A differential spinal block may be used. The concept of a differential lumbar spinal with local anesthetics is to inject into the CSF first a placebo such as normal saline, then a dilute, weak strength local anesthetic such as isobaric 0.5% procaine (or an appropriate concentration of a different local anesthetic), which is thought to primarily block sympathetic fibers. The volume required will vary depending upon the site of pain, but 2 – 3 ml is usually adequate. This is to be followed by 1.0% procaine for sensory block and 2% procaine for motor block. The entire procedure is preferably done via an indwelling catheter with the patient lying on his back.

If the patient responds to the placebo the thought is that the pain is primarily of psychogenic origin. It must however be remembered that 30% – 40% of all patients will be placebo responders. Therefore one should not overinterpret the results of a single diagnostic block. The response to a placebo injection in any patient may be variable, i.e., they may or may not have pain relief with any injection. In addition, the placebo response is usually short lived in patients with a true organic cause for their pain. If one sees a consistent response to placebo injections of significant durations this suggests strongly that further investigation with nerve block therapy is no longer indicated.

If the patient responds to the dilute (0.5% procaine) solution then the assumption is that there is a high sympathetic nervous system component to the discomfort. 1.0% procaine will block sensory nerves. If the patient has no response to 2% procaine, which produces both sensory and motor block, pain of central origin or of a psychological nature must be considered. It would be foolhardy to proceed with peripheral procedures, be they neurosurgery or destructive neurolytic nerve blocks, in such a case.

The same approach could be carried out in the epidural space with a catheter in place. In this case concentrations of 0%, 0.5%, 1.0%, and 2.0% lidocaine provide similar information to that described above.

Some centers have used selective epidural analgesia with a narcotic as the test substance. For example, 1 μg/kg of fentanyl mixed with 5 ml of saline in the epidural space will rapidly diffuse through the dura and block pain receptors in the substantia gelatinosa of the spinal cord. This amount of fentanyl will not produce a high enough blood level to cause any significant systemic effects. The patient will not be unaware of any peripheral sensations, as he would be when local anesthetics are used as described above. The attainment of pain relief would indicate that the painful source is at a point peripheral to the spinal cord.

Suggested reading

Cherry DA, Gourlay GK, McLachlan M et al. (1985) Diagnostic epidural opioid blockade and chronic pain: preliminary report. Pain 21:143

Ramamurthy S, Winnie AP (1985) Regional anesthetic techniques for pain relief. Semin Anaesth 4:237

Sanders SH, McKeel NL, Hare BD (1984) Relationship between psychopathology and graduated spinal block findings in chronic pain patients. Pain 19:367

Winnie AP, Ramamurthy S, Durrani Z (1974) Diagnostic and therapeutic nerve blocks: recent advances in techniques. Adv Neurol 4:455

A word of caution about the above is required. It must be remembered that any intervention by a physician has a very positive psychological effect on the patient. A simplistic interpretation of the response to any single peripheral procedure or set of procedures (i.e., differential spinal) should be avoided, especially if these are to lead to either surgical interventions or potentially hazardous block procedures.

There are many (including the authors) who question the value of the above procedures since the differential blocking effects of local anesthetics are not as sharply defined as the above suggests. Recent evidence concerning the various intraspinal sites of action of local anesthetics with differing lipid solubility coefficients severely question the entire concept of differential block. We therefore prefer the following scheme when trying to differentiate between various types of thoraco-abdominal pain:

Step 1. – The patient is given a spinal anesthetic to the T4 level. If pain is not blocked at this point this indicates either a central somatic or a psychogenic etiology and militates against additional nerve blocking procedures. An exception to this could be pain involving vagal afferents only, though such pain is extremely rare. If the pain is blocked then one proceeds with step 2 the next day.

Step 2. – A somatic nerve block, usually in the form of intercostal blocks at the angle of the rib posteriorly, is performed in order to rule out a somatic component. For the upper abdomen intercostal nerves 6 through 10 are blocked. For the lower abdomen blocks include intercostal nerves 11 and 12. If the results are positive this indicates that the problem is one primarily involving structures innervated by somatic nerve branches. By blocking individual groups of intercostal nerves the specific area of pain is defined. Definitive therapy in the form of permanent blocks, surgery, medical treatment, etc. can then be more rationally administered.

Step 3. – If the somatic nerve blocks are ineffective in relieving pain then a diagnostic celiac plexus block is done, which should confirm that pain is of visceral origin. This in turn may lead to further medical and/or surgical intervention, depending upon the nature and severity of the pain. A series of epidural blocks done in the lower thoracic region, i.e., at the T10 level, in order to block the sympathetic preganglionic fibers to the splanchnic area could provide the same information as the technically more difficult celiac plexus block in many patients. If there is any question that the vagal afferents might be involved, a celiac plexus block should be done.

Vague abdominal visceral pain is almost always amenable to appropriate medical workup and therapy. A very rare circumstance indeed would be the use of a neurolytic block of the celiac plexus for the treatment of vague abdominal pain.

Special pain problems

Cancer pain – the technique of spinal neurolysis

Subarachnoid alcohol

Subarachnoid alcohol injection is best used for the management of unilateral somatic pain, in particular pain secondary to metastases to bones or peripheral soft tissue with somatic nerve irritation. It must be remembered that the periosteum of the bone has its own innervation which may or may not be related to the specific skin dermatome area under which it lies. For example, the ribs are innervated segmentally so that the seventh rib has its major innervation from the seventh thoracic nerve although the periosteum may also receive some minor innervation from T6. On the other hand, a small area of bone in the pelvis might have as many as three or four different nerve roots supplying sensation to it. The bony sclerotomal innervation must be understood so that the appropriate nerves are identified.

Also, since the procedure involves the deposition of alcohol in the CSF surrounding the dorsal rootlets of spinal nerves, the origin of these nerves in relation to the bony spinal canal should be understood. For example, if one wanted to anesthetize the T8 and T9 nerves it must be remembered that the dorsal rootlets of these nerves originate two interspaces higher, in other words at T6 and T7. Similarly, all of the lumbar and sacral nerves have their origins at the terminal portions of the cord from T10 to L1.

If there is uncertainty whether the neurolytic procedure will provide adequate analgesia, it is wise to start with a hypobaric spinal using the exact same technique. In this case a small amount of hypobaric tetracaine, usually 1 – 2 mg in 1 – 2 ml of sterile water for injection, will give a short-lived temporary analgesia similar to that which would be obtained with alcohol. If this proves satisfactory to the patient then the neurolytic procedure should be done the next day.

With the anatomy in mind the procedure is as follows: the patient is placed on an operating table and turned to the 45° prone position with the painful side up. The site of the injection should be raised either by bending the operating room table or by having the patient lie on a foam pillow to give a distinct curve to the spinal cord, so that the site of injection is uppermost. A 10-cm 22 or 20 gauge spinal needle is inserted into the subarachnoid space. It must be remembered that all injections will be in either the cervical or the thoracic region and over the substance of the spinal cord, so particular care must be taken not to thrust the needle ahead too rapidly. Once the arachnoid is pierced and a clear flow of CSF appears, 0.25 ml of absolute alcohol is teased in using a 1-ml tuberculin syringe. The patient will have been told previously that he might experience a short lived (15 s) paresthesia which might be quite severe. He is to report to the operator where the paresthesia is without moving. If the paresthesia is to the correct anatomic site the definitive injection is carried out. If the paresthesia is either below or above the correct site and remembering that alcohol is hypobaric (specific gravity of 0.8 compared with 1.006 for CSF), the table is manipulated so as the alcohol will flow in either a cranial or a caudad direction. A second subarachnoid puncture should be done at the appropriate level in case of marked disparity between the initial paresthesia and the area of pain.

Absolute alcohol is then injected slowly, about 0.25 – 0.5 ml per minute, until the final volume is deposited. The total volume required depends upon the number of dermatomes that one wishes to block and the general state of the patient (a debilitated patient requiring less drug than one who is well hydrated and less debilitated). Usually 2 – 3 ml alcohol is required to anesthetize a three to five dermatome area in the mid-thoracic region. As the alcohol is being injected its effects on skin sensation are tested by pinprick. It is very common to see the initial injection of 3 ml alcohol provide as much as a 12 – 14 dermatome spread of analgesia, which will rapidly diminish.

The patient is maintained on the operating room table in the same position for about 20 min to allow the alcohol to "fix" to the neural tissue and decrease migration to other parts of the subarachnoid space. After 20 min the patient is put on his back and observed for a few hours in this position. By the next morning he should be able to ambulate with assistance, general physical condition permitting.

When correctly done this procedure will provide a chemical dorsal root rhizotomy which will last anywhere from 2 to 6 months or longer. Unfortunately that is the average and the authors have seen cases in which pain has returned within 48–72 h, probably due to incomplete neurolysis. The procedure is then repeated.

After a correctly performed subarachnoid neurolytic block significant improvement of the patient's objective condition (reduced need for analgesics, improved appetite and sleeping pattern, etc.) can be observed in the majority of cases. When asked, patients frequently deny improvement as mental depression, side effects, narcotic addiction, etc. contribute considerably to the general condition and affect the state of well-being. In various published materials the results have been classified as good in approximately 50 % – 60 %, fair in 20 % – 30 % and poor in 15 % – 20 %.

Whenever a neurolytic agent such as alcohol is injected into the central nervous system the possibility of untoward sequelae always exists. Paresis and/or rectal and urinary dysfunction are reported in 2 % – 25 % of cases, sensory loss in 1 % to 10 %, and paresthesia/neuritis in 0.3 % – 3.4 %. Sphincter dysfunction is chiefly associated with lumbosacral blocks. The complications are usually transient but fatalities and permanent neurologic sequelae are reported.

Suggested reading

Bonica JJ (1958) Diagnostic and therapeutic blocks: a reappraisal based on 15 years' experience. Anesth Analg 37:58

Dogliotti AM (1931) Traitement des syndromes douloureux de la pèriphèrie par l'alcoolisation subarachnoidienne. Presse Med 67:11

Drechsel, U. (1984) Treatment of cancer pain with neurolytic agents. Recent Results Cancer Res 89:137

Dwyer B, Gibb D (1980) Chronic pain and neurolytic neural blockade. In: Cousins MJ, Bridenbaugh PO (eds) Neural blockade in clinical anesthesia and management of pain. J.B. Lippincott, Philadelphia, p 637

Gerbershagen HU, Baar HA, Kreuscher H (1972) Langzeitnervenblockaden zur Behandlung schwerer Schmerzzust)84(nde»I. Die intrathecale Injektion von Neurolytica. Der Anaesthesist 21:112

Greenhill JP (1947) Sympathectomy and intraspinal alcohol injections for the relief of pelvic pain. Br Med J II:859

Hay RC (1962) Subarachnoid alcohol block in the control of intractable pain: report of results in 252 patients. Anesth Analg 41:12

Ischia S, Luzzani A, Ischia A et al. (1984) Subarachnoid neurolytic block (L5-S1) and unilateral percutaneous cervical cordotomy in the treatment of pain secondary to pelvic malignant disease. Pain 20:139

Kuzucu EY, Derrick WS, Wilber SA (1966) Control of intractable pain with subarachnoid alcohol block. JAMA 195:541

Maher R, Mehta M (1977) Spinal (intrathecal) and extradural analgesia. In: Lipton S (ed) Persistent pain: modern methods of treatment, vol 1. Academic Press, London, p 61

Mehta M (1981) Improvements in spinal injection treatment for cancer pain. In: Lipton S, Miles J (eds) Persistent pain: modern methods of treatment, vol. 3. Academic Press, London, p 265

Murphy TM (1983) Complications of neurolytic blocks. In: Orkin FK, Cooperman LH (eds) Complications in anesthesiology. J.B. Lippincott, Philadelphia, p 117

Swerdlow M (1982) Spinal and peripheral neurolysis for managing Pancoast syndrome. In: Bonica JJ, Ventafridda V, Pagni CA (eds) Management of superior pulmonary sulcus syndrome (Pancoast syndrome). Advances in pain research and therapy, Vol 4. Raven Press, New York, p 135

Swerdlow M (1983) Intrathecal and extradural block in pain relief. In: Swerdlow M (ed) Relief of intractable pain. Elsevier Scientific, Amsterdam, p 177

Ventafridda V, Spreafico R (1974) Subarachnoid saline perfusion. Adv Neurol 4:477

Subarachnoid phenol

Some authors recommend using a hyperbaric phenol solution, i.e., 6% – 10% phenol dissolved in glycerin, instead of the hypobaric alcohol. They suggest that the results are somewhat better and the incidence of postoperative neuritis less. However, the incidence of complications related to the vascular or thrombogenic effects of phenol seems worthy of mention. As a result of such complications we consider that subarachnoid neurolytic blocks are preferably performed with alcohol.

If heavy phenol were to be used the procedure would be identical to that described above except that the patient would be turned with the painful side down, leaning backward. Many patients cannot tolerate this position without additional analgesics which tend to obscure the immediate results of the injection.

The total dose of phenol usually ranges from 0.5 to 1.0 ml depending chiefly on the distribution of the patient's pain.

Being aware of the risk of sphincter dysfunction, heavy phenol solutions can be used with caution for the treatment of perineal and pelvic pain. In such a case lumbar puncture is performed at L5 – S1 with the patient in the sitting position. For bilateral pain 0.5 – 0.7 ml phenol, 7.5% – 15% in glycerin, is injected slowly (0.1 ml/5 min) with the patient leaned backward to about 45° to the table and supported in this position by an assistant. For a unilateral block the patient is lowered to 45° with the table and the upper part of the body is rotated toward the painful side. After completion of the injection the patient is maintained in the appropriate position for 20 min to 3 h.

Suggested reading

Brown AS (1981) Current views on the use of nerve blocking in the relief of chronic pain. In: Swerdlow M et al. (eds) Current status of modern therapy, vol 6. The therapy of pain. MTP Press, Lancaster, p 127

Dwyer B, Gibb D (1980) Chronic pain and neurolytic neural blockade. In: Cousins MJ, Bridenbaugh PO (eds) Neural blockade in clinical anesthesia and management of pain. JB Lippincott, Philadelphia, p 637

Edwards WT, Burney RG, Peeters-Asdourian C (1985) Development of segmental tonic – clonic activity following subarachnoid phenol injection. Reg Anesth 10:91

Gerbershagen HU, Baar HA, Kreuscher H (1972) Langzeitnervenblockaden zur Behandlung schwerer Schmerzzustände 1. Die intrathecale Injektion von Neurolytica. Der Anaesthesist 21:112

Swerdlow M (1980) Complications of neurolytic neural blockade. In: Cousins MJ, Bridenbaugh PO (eds) Neural blockade in clinical anesthesia and management of pain. JB Lippincott, Philadelphia, p 543

Swerdlow M (1983) Intrathecal and extradural block in pain relief. In: Swerdlow M, (ed) Relief of intractable pain. Elsevier Scientific, Amsterdam, p 177.

Epidural phenol

Subarachnoid neurolysis will provide satisfactory results and a reasonably low complication rate. Some authors, however, believe that epidural neurolysis is more satisfactory in the cervical and upper thoracic region. For this purpose a segmental technique is used and a catheter introduced 2 – 3 cm. Solutions of 6% – 7.5% phenol in water or glycerin are used in volumes ranging from 1 to 5 ml. Following the injection of phenol in glycerin, pain disappears over 5 – 10 minutes. For the next 24 – 48 h attacks of severe pain may still occur but they become less frequent with time and eventually disappear.

Suggested reading

Brown AS (1981) Current views on the use of nerve blocking in the relief of chronic pain. In: Swerdlow M et al.(eds) Current status of modern therapy, vol 6. The therapy of pain. MTP Press, Lancaster, p 116

Coombs DW (1985) Potential hazards of transcatheter serial epidural phenol neurolysis. Anesth Analg 64:1205

Transsacral neurolytic block

Perineal pain secondary to carcinomas in the pelvic cavity may occur in inoperable cases or following attempts at resection. The pain tends to be constant and is frequently very intense. The patients are typically unable to sit because of aggravation of the pain.

Intrathecal neurolysis is difficult to accomplish without affecting control of the bladder and/or rectum. Perineal sensory innervation is predominantly a function of the S4 spinal nerve. By selective neurolysis of this and/or other appropriate sacral nerve(s) a significant reduction in the intensity of the pain can be obtained without any untoward effects on the patients' ability to control the rectal and urinary sphincters.

The technique of transsacral (sacral paravertebral) block has been described on p 141. In patients with perineal pain secondary to cancer it is recommended that one proceeds in the following order:

1. Unilateral or bilateral transsacral block of S4 is induced by 2 – 4 ml of 0.5% bupivacaine dependent on the localization of the pain.

2. Evaluation of the pain relief and the patients' ability to control the rectal and urinary sphincters can be made 20 min thereafter.

3. In case of unsatisfactory pain relief, additional sacral nerves can be blocked with bupivacaine but no more than three or four nerves should be blocked at the same session.

4. When mapping of the appropriate sacral nerves responsible for propagation has been carried out and one has made certain that these nerves are not involved in the control of the sphincters, neurolytic block with 2 – 3 ml of 6% phenol in water is performed. The number of nerves subject to neurolysis should be kept to a minimum and additional blocks performed at a subsequent session if necessary.

5. Frequently the duration of pain relief is only about 1 week, so the patient should be seen at this time and receive a second injection if necessary. Duration of analgesia varies considerably so one might have to repeat injections every month or so.

The technique is easy to perform and requires minimal facilities. Complications are few and the technique can be used on an outpatient basis

Suggested reading

Robertson DH (1983) Transsacral neurolytic nerve block. An alternative approach to intractable perineal pain. Br J Anaesth 55:873

Celiac plexus block for cancer pain or chronic pancreatitis

The technique for celiac plexus block has been described on p 138. The block should be carried out with a local anesthetic prior to the use of neurolytic agents to ascertain its efficacy for pain relief in these conditions. If the local anesthetic block provides the desired results, the neurolytic procedure is performed bilaterally the next day. Since the alcohol must be precisely placed, X-ray verification of the position of the needle tips is beneficial. The transverse process and body of the L1 vertebra are located and the needles advanced trans-crurally 2 cm beyond and anterior to the lateral border of the body into the retroperitoneal space on both sides. This position should be verified by fluoroscopy. Between 15 and 30 ml of 50% alcohol is then injected through the needles on each side. Injection frequently causes rather severe visceral pain in the upper abdomen. This can to some extent be prevented by pre-injection of 5 – 10 ml of 0.25% bupivacaine through each needle. Alcohol injection is done 5 min thereafter.

An alternative technique which is being used more frequently is to perform the block with only one needle placed on the left. After X-ray verification of needle tip position 15 – 30 cc of absolute alcohol or larger volumes of 50% alcohol are injected.

The patient is maintained prone for several minutes and then returned carefully to his back, monitoring blood pressure constantly since significant hypotension might occur with movement. Blood pressure monitoring is continued until the next day and the patient is watched very carefully. Ambulation should be done with assistance until it is determined that postural hypotension does not occur.

When used for relief of pain secondary to cancer of the stomach, liver, pancreas, gallbladder, bowel, and kidneys results have been reported to be good to excellent in 85% – 98%. In pain secondary to chronic pancreatitis, however, the results are such poorer.

The duration of pain relief is often life-long for patients with cancer but the block must occasionally be repeated. In chronic pancreatitis a mean duration of 2 months has been reported.

Since the results are gratifying in the cancer patient, we suggest that the indications for neurolytic plexus block for cancer are very strong. In contrast are the relatively poor results, the need for frequent blocks, and the concomitant psychological problems that occur in patients with pain from chronic pancreatitis, especially when due to alcoholism.

Complications

In almost all cases a transient postural hypotension occurs which sometimes requires infusion of crystalloids or colloids. Extremely rare cases of paraplegia, loss of ejaculation or pleural effusion have been reported. Radiologic control of needle position is therefore strongly advocated.

Suggested reading

Bridenbaugh LD, Moore DC, Campbell DD (1964) Management of upper abdominal cancer pain. JAMA 190:877

Gorbitz C, Leavens ME (1971) Alcohol block of the coeliac plexus for control of upper abdominal pain caused by cancer and pancreatitis. J Neurosurg 34:575

Jones J, Gough D (1977) Aspects of treatment. Coeliac plexus block with alcohol for relief of upper abdominal pain due to cancer. Ann R Coll Surg Engl 58:46

Leung JWC, Bowenwright M, Aveling W et al. (1983) Coeliac plexus block for pain in pancreatic cancer and chronic pancreatitis. Br J Surg 70:730

Moore DC (1979) Coeliac (splanchnic) plexus block with alcohol for cancer pain of upper intraabdominal viscera. In: Bonica JJ, Ventafridda V, (eds) Advances in pain research and therapy, vol 2. Raven Press, New York, p 357

Owitz S, Koppolu S (1983) Celiac plexus block: an overview. Mt Sinai J Med 50:486

Thompson GE, Moore DC, Bridenbaugh LD et al. (1977) Abdominal pain and alcohol celiac plexus nerve block. Anesth Analg 56:1

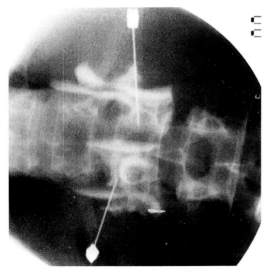

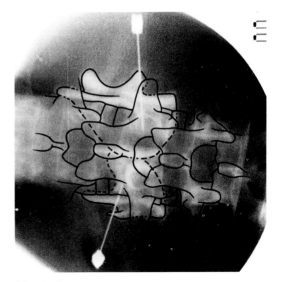

Fig. 4.1a. Celiac plexus block. A-P view of the needles placed at the upper (right side) and middle (left side) third of the L₁ vertebral body. The tip of the left and right needles are located approximately 2.0 and 1.5 cm ventral to the anterior aspect of the vertebral body, respectively. Despite this placement of needles the spread of the contrast reveals that the tips are located retrocrurally. However, the dye emerges ventrally along the celiac axis.

Fig. 4.1b.

In the operating room the anesthesiologist might stimulate the surgeons to perform chemical splanchnicectomy with phenol intraoperatively in patients with unresectable carcinoma of the pancreas.

Suggested reading

Gardner AMN, Solomou G (1984) Relief of the pain of unresectable carcinoma of pancreas by chemical splanchnicectomy during laparotomy. Ann R Coll Surg Engl 66:409

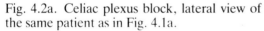

Fig. 4.2a. Celiac plexus block, lateral view of the same patient as in Fig. 4.1a.

Fig. 4.2b.

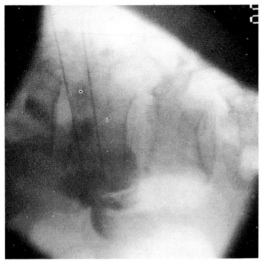

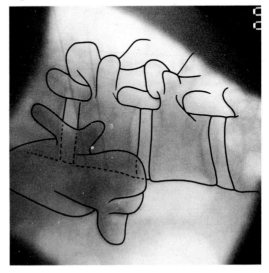

175

Cancer pain – the use of epidural opioids

The advantage of epidural opioid analgesia over epidurally administered local anesthetics is that nociceptive input to the central nervous system is blocked selectively. Thus proprioceptive, motor and sympathetic nerve fibers are not affected so that the patient can experience normal skin sensation. Motor function and the circulatory system are not affected.

Through epidural administration of opioids, pain resulting from a variety of causes, including cancer, can be controlled. Our present knowledge is limited and the recommendations given below might be subject to changes within the near future.

For treatment of severe cancer pain the method can be used for hospitalized or ambulatory patients. In general, the results have been favorable but it has been pointed out that different types of cancer pain respond differently, even when present in the same patient. Continuous somatic pain responds very favorably, while continuous visceral pain, intermittent somatic pain, and continuous neurogenic pain are less affected. Intermittent visceral or neurogenic pain as well as cutaneous pain is not alleviated by epidural opioids. For these types of pain, subarachnoid or celiac neurolytic blocks should be applied when peroral analgesics are no longer effective.

Irrespective of the dermatomal level of pain a lumbar epidural administration suffices. A segmental technique, with its associated risks, results in the same intensity and duration of pain relief as lumbar administration. For long-term treatment the epidural catheter should be tunneled subcutaneously from the puncture site ventrally toward the lower portion of the rib cage. Tunneling along the spine should be avoided as it is associated with a considerably higher incidence of catheter dislocations. Preferably implantable injection ports should be used to allow the patient the comfort of showering or taking a bath. These are expensive, however, and in many cases one can manage with percutaneous catheters firmly secured with Steristrip or Tegaderm.

Intermittent injections of preservative-free morphine are most commonly used. As a rule, the treatment starts with a dose of 2 – 4 mg, two to four times a day. In the event of unsatisfactory results, the dose is increased until an optimal effect is achieved without intolerable side effects.

Continuous infusion of opioids has been shown to have certain advantages over intermittent injections such as a reduced need for opioids, a constant level of analgesia, greater convenience for patients and staff, and a lower incidence of catheter-related complications. The incidence of conventional side-effects is reported to be much lower. A continuous infusion can be administered by means of implantable or externally worn pumps. A variety of these devices are available. Up till now they have one common property – a high price – which makes it necessary to limit their use to patients with a reasonably long life-expectancy.

It is still the case that only limited data exist on what is an adequate dosage of constantly injected morphine in the epidural space. An initial daily consumption of 4 mg might rise to more than 100 mg. By continuous-plus-on-demand infusion epidurally, the daily morphine consumption can be kept much lower.

Irrespective of the technique of administration, tachyphylaxis occurs and the dosages must be increased in order to maintain the patient in a reasonable pain-free condition. Equipotent doses of other opioids may be given but the vast majority of our experience today is from patients given morphine.

One of the major advantages with epidural morphine administration is that the patient can be nursed at home in a reasonably

pain-free state. For insertion of the catheter and the initial titration of the dosage
regimen the patient should be hospitalized
overnight. In most cases it is possible to dis-
charge the patient on the next morning provided that he, his wife, or the district nurse
has learned how to manage opioid administration. We see our patients with percutaneous catheters at the pain clinic once
a week, while patients with implanted delivery systems can be seen less frequently.

It seems as if patients with cancer pain provide a very favorable risk-benefit ratio,
especially those already tolerant to parenteral opioids. In patients with continuous somatic pain the results are excellent
provided the dosage of opioids is correctly
titrated. Respiratory depression has not
been reported and urinary problems, itching, and nausea are rare, especially when
continuous or continuous-plus-on-demand
infusion is employed. However, concomitant administration of opioids epidurally
and parenterally should preferably be
avoided.

Despite the large number of patients
treated in this way, systematic investigations are scarce. The ideal treatment regimen has most likely not yet been found
and a word of caution against uncritical use
of this method is therefore issued.

Suggested reading

Ali NMK, Hanna N (1985) Long-term percutaneous epidural catheteri-
zation for cancer pain. Reg Anesth 10:32

Arnèr S, Arnèr B (1985) Differential effects of epidural morphine in the
treatment of cancer-related pain. Acta Anaesthesiol Scand 29:32

Auld AW, Maki-Jokela A, Murdoch DM (1985) Intraspinal narcotic
analgesia in the treatment of chronic pain. Spine 10:777

Carl P, Crawford ME, Ravlo O et al. (1986) Long-term treatment with
epidural opioids. A retrospective study comprising 150 patients
treated with morphine chloride and buprenorphine. Anaesthesia 41:32

Chrubasik J (1985) Spinal infusion of opiates and somatostatin.
Fresenius Foundation, Verlag Hygieneplan, Oberursel FRG

Coombs DW (1986) Management of chronic pain by epidural and
intrathecal opioids: newer drugs and delivery systems. Int Anesthesiol
Clin 24:59

Cousins MJ, Mather LE (1984) Intrathecal epidural administration of
opioids. Anesthesiology 61:276

Crawford ME, Andersen G, Augustenborg J et al (1983) Pain treatment
on outpatient basis utilizing extradural opiates. A Danish multicentre
study comprising 105 patients. Pain 16:41

Krames ES, Gershow J, Glassberg A et al (1985) Continuous infusion of
spinally administered narcotics for relief of pain due to malignant
disorders. Cancer 56:696

Max MB, Inturrisi CE, Kaiko RF (1985) Epidural and intrathecal
opiates: cerebrospinal fluid and plasma profiles in patients with
chronic cancer pain. Clin Pharmacol Ther 38:631

Michon F, Des Mesnards VG, Girard M et al (1985) Long-term peridural
morphine analgesia in neoplastic and vascular pathology. Cah
Anesthesiol 33:39

Rawal N, Sjöstrand UH (1986) Clinical application of epidural and
intrathecal opioids for pain management. Int Anesthesiol Clin 24:43

Wang JK (1985) Intrathecal morphine for intractable pain secondary to
cancer of pelvic organs. Pain 21:99

Acute abdominal pain

There are several disease states in which acute pain in the abdomen can be alleviated while the underlying basic pathology is being treated. These include acute pancreatitis, biliary colic, and ureteral colic.

One of the major pathologic features of acute pancreatitis is pain. This may be so severe as to cause a rigid abdomen and associated pulmonary dysfunction. It is not unusual to have to narcotize the patient heavily while treating the underlying pathology.

Alternatives to the use of parenteral narcotics are blocks of the celiac plexus or splanchnic nerves and, more preferably, a continuous segmental epidural. The epidural should be done in the low thoracic area to anesthetize the preganglionic fibers to the celiac plexus. Bupivacaine, in a volume of 6 – 10 ml of 0.5% solution, injected at the T10 interspace via an epidural catheter, will provide satisfactory analgesia and perhaps diminish the associated biliary duct spasm, which in many cases is thought to be a major pathophysiologic feature of the disease. The block is continued by injections of 3 – 5 ml every second hour (or by the corresponding dose given as constant infusion) for several days, the precise duration depending on the course of the disease. It seems as if this form of pain therapy helps produce a more rapid resolution of the disease.

The same logic applies to the treatment of acute biliary colic where not only can pain be relieved but the possibility exists that smaller gallstones may be passed. According to our experience a single splanchnic nerve or celiac plexus block is sufficient to relieve most patients from their discomfort and only rarely should it be necessary to apply continuous techniques. To the best of our knowledge there are no data concerning whether the use of epidural analgesia or celiac blocks indeed shorten the course of acute biliary colic. There is, however, at least one report indicating that the use of continuous epidural analgesia has helped patients pass ureteral calculi that have otherwise been impacted somewhere along the course of the ureter. This therapy was used in conjunction with hydration of the patients with a rather good success rate.

As in the case of acute biliary colic, a single splanchnic or celiac block usually suffices to relieve the often agonizing pain in patients with acute renal colic. Any block may be technically difficult to perform in these patients, as one of the characteristic features of acute renal colic is that the patients constantly move around.

Suggested reading

Dale WA (1952) Splanchnic block in the treatment of acute pancreatitis. Surgery 32:605

Howard JM, Milford MT, DeBakey ME (1952) The significance of the sympathetic nervous system in acute cholecystitis. Surgery 32:251

Lundskog O, Baar HA, Ahlgren J (1973) 10 Jahre Erfahrung mit der Blockadetherapie. Anaesthesiol Wiederbelebung 73:27

Tassonyi E, Kun M, Rozsa I et al. (1981) Epidural block in the treatment of acute pancreatitis. Reg Anesth 6:8

Bladder pain

The "painful contracted bladder" is a consequence of, for example, radiation, chronic infection, calculi, interstitial cystitis, or neurologic injury or disease. The symptoms usually consist of urgency, frequency and pain on urination associated with a reduced bladder capacity and incontinence. Often patients are unable to partake in normal physical or social activities and become "bladder cripples."

In individual cases specific therapy should of course be instituted. Not infrequently this therapy does not relieve the patient from his main complaint: the painful contracted bladder. Surgical therapy that has been tried includes denervation or rhizotomy, with improvement in approximately 50% of cases. Extensive palliative procedures such as enterocystoplasty result in up to 65% satisfactory results but carry a certain mortality and a significant complication rate.

Bladder dysfunction has been treated by transsacral nerve blocks for many decades. As such a block is very easily performed and carries very little risk, it should be remembered for patients with bladder pain.

The technique of transsacral (sacral paravertebral) block has been described on p 141. The following procedure is recommended:

1. A right S3 transsacral nerve block is performed using 2 – 4 ml 0.5% bupivacaine.

2. If there is no subjective improvement within 24 h a left S3 block is performed.

3. Additional blocks of the adjacent sacral nerves may sometimes be performed after observation periods of 24 h following the preceding block. Next to S3, S2 seems to be the nerve most frequently involved in bladder pain.

4. When the correct sacral nerve has been identified one might go ahead with either repeat blocks with local anesthetics or neurolytic blocks. The choice depends on the severity of the underlying disease and the symptoms.

5. Repeat blocks with local anesthetics may be given every second day for four or five times. If no long-lasting improvement ensues, one should go ahead with neurolytic block with 6% phenol in water, 1.5 – 2 ml per nerve. Occasionally one might have to repeat the block after one to several weeks.

Considering that the very simple transsacral neurolysis is reported to have approximately the same success rate as comprehensive surgical procedures in relieving the patient's pain, it seems reasonable that transsacral nerve blocks should be tried in appropriate patients.

Suggested reading

Gerbershagen HU, Frohneberg DH, Panhans Ch et al. (1984) Transsacral block. In: van Kleef JW, Burm AGL, Spierdijk J (eds) Current concepts in regional anaesthesia. Proceeding of the second general meeting of the European Society of Regional Anaesthesia. Martinus Nijhoff, The Hague, p 23.

Simon DL, Carron H, Rowlingson JC (1982) Treatment of bladder pain with transsacral nerve block. Anesth Analg 61:46

Chest wall trauma and fractured ribs

The pain secondary to trauma of the chest wall is often easily relieved by nerve blocking procedures.

For limited areas of discomfort, such as might occur after fractures of one to three ribs, repeated intercostal injections may be used. Injections should include intercostal spaces cephalad and caudad to the fractured ribs to block the overlap of innervation from adjacent segments. Long-acting local anesthetics, such as 0.5% bupivacaine with adrenaline, will provide up to 8 – 10 h of pain relief.

In order to save the patient from repeated annoying reinjections, subsequent blocks should be performed while the previous one is still in effect. For the average simple fractured rib these injections need to be repeated for about 2 days. In more extensive cases the analgesia may be continued from 7 to as many as 12 days.

Repetition of blocks over a long period or in multitraumatized patients might be extremely inconvenient for the patient as well as for support personnel. Alternative blocking techniques therefore have to be considered.

Continuous intercostal blocks can be accomplished after insertion of epidural catheters in the appropriate intercostal spaces. In order to be effective they must be properly secured and injected every eighth hour with 3 ml of 0.5% bupivacaine with adrenaline through a bacterial filter. Satisfactory results have also been reported when a single-catheter technique has been utilized. This may be due to spread of the local anesthetic within the fracture hematoma or to disruption of the normal anatomy. The appropriate dose will be initially 20 ml of 0.5% bupivacaine with adrenaline followed by 10 ml every eighth hour. Our results with this technique have been marginal. Not all patients obtained an appropriate level of analgesia. The intrapleural catheter technique for intercostal blocks has been described on p 134.

Another alternative, especially for pain involving both sides, is a continuous thoracic epidural block with either local anesthetics or opioids. This technique is described on p 110.

In patients with flail chest epidural analgesia has in many cases been successful in replacing the more conventional endotracheal intubation – controlled ventilation – parenteral narcotic regime. It appears that the epidural will not only provide pain relief but also allow for maintenance of almost normal pulmonary function.

Suggested reading

Dittmann M, Ferstl A, Wolfe G (1975) Epidural analgesia for the treatment of multiple rib fractures. Eur J Intensive Care Med 1:71

Gibbons J, James O, Quail A (1973) Management of 130 cases of chest injury with respiratory failure. Br J Anaesth 45:1130

Möller-Pedersen W, Schulze S, Höier-Madsen K et al. (1983) Air-flow meter assessment of the effect of intercostal nerve blockade on respiratory function in rib fractures. Acta Chir Scand 149:119

O'Kelley E, Garry B (1981) Continuous pain relief for multiple fractured ribs. Br J Anaesth 53:989

Rankin APN, Comber REH (1984) Management of fifty cases of chest injury with a regimen of epidural bupivacaine and morphine. Anaesth Intens Care 12:311

Shackford JR, Smith DE, Zarins CK et al (1976) Management of flail chest. A comparison of ventilatory and non-ventilatory treatment. Am J Surg 132:759

Trinkel JR, Richardson JD, Franz JL et al (1975) Management of flail chest without mechanical ventilation. Ann Thorac Surg 19:355

Worthley LIG (1985) Thoracic epidural in the management of chest trauma. A study of 161 cases. Intensive Care Med 11:312

Herpes zoster and postherpetic neuralgia

Herpes zoster is characterized by radicular pain, which is sometimes very severe, vesicular cutaneous eruptions, and less often sensory loss or motor palsies. The pathology includes inflammation of the dorsal root or cranial nerve ganglia with extension into the posterior horn of the spinal cord.

There is a prodromal period of 3 – 4 days of itching or burning sensations involving one or several dermatomes after which vesicular lesions erupt, confirming the diagnosis.

In most cases the disease is self-limited and segmental pain lasts for 1 – 4 weeks. However, the pain may persist as a postherpetic neuralgia, especially in the aged or debilitated patient. Postherpetic neuralgia characteristically has two features: (a) a constant, often severe, radicular pain, and (b) dysesthesia, which means that the patient is extremely sensitive to the slightest touch to the affected skin area. The incidence of postherpetic neuralgia has been reported to be 7% – 50% of cases. In most cases the symptoms fade out after months to years but they occasionally persist.

There is some evidence that sympathetic nerve blocks done at the appropriate level early in the course of the disease not only alleviate the pain and shorten the skin manifestations of the acute process, but also protects the patient from postherpetic neuralgia. The treatment is given every second day employing 0.25% bupivacaine, with or without adrenaline. In a typical case pain relief occurs within 10 – 15 min and lasts for up to 12 h. Shorter lasting painrelief indicates an unsuccessful outcome of this treatment. Statements can be found in the literature suggesting that when sympathetic nerve blocks are done early in the course (within 2 weeks), the incidence of postherpetic neuralgia will be almost nil.

Since the majority of the sympathetic outflow can be interrupted by intercostal or paravertebral blocks a series of these blocks should be instituted as early as chest or abdominal wall herpes zoster is diagnosed. In the upper thoracic area (as well as for facial or the less common brachial locations) stellate ganglion blocks are indicated. Single injection epidural blocks will serve the same purpose, especially in the rare instance of bilateral involvement.

As the disease progresses into the postherpetic neuralgia phase the efficacy of blocks decreases although a 50% success rate has been reported. In resistant cases a subcutaneous infiltration of the painful area with, for example, 30 ml of 0.25% bupivacaine with adrenaline mixed with 40 – 80 mg methylprednisolone has been advocated. In many cases therapy is unsuccessful and in fact even central nervous system destructive procedures such as rhizotomies or cordotomies have failed to provide relief in chronic cases. Therefore nerve block procedures should be done as early in the course of the disease as possible.

Recently some investigators have treated the pain of postherpetic neuralgia with epidural narcotic injections with reported success.

Since the disease is almost always self-limiting, although its course may be protracted, the use of neurodestructive or neurolytic blocking techniques is not indicated.

Suggested reading

Colding A (1973) Treatment of pain: organization of a pain clinic: treatment of acute herpes zoster. Proc R Soc Med 66:541

Dan K, Higa K, Tanaka K et al. (1983) Herpetic pain and cellular immunity. In: Yokota T, Dubner R,(eds) Current topics in pain research and therapy. Proceedings of the international symposium on pain. Kyoto, Dec 12–13, 1982. Excerpta Medica, Amsterdam, p 293

Forrest JB (1978) Management of chronic dorsal root pain with epidural steroid. Can Anaesth Soc J 25:218

Lipton S (1979) Relief of pain in clinical practice. Blackwell Scientific, Oxford, p 231.

Milligan NS, Nash TP (1985) Treatment of post-herpetic neuralgia. A review of 77 consecutive cases. Pain 23:381

Ramamurthy S, Winnie AP (1985) Regional anesthetic techniques for pain relief. Semin Anesth 4:237

Selander D, Nordin P (1986) Early epidural or sympathetic block cures herpes zoster and prevents post-herpetic neuralgia. In: Rosberg B (ed) Proceedings from ESRA, Malmö, 1986.

Winnie AP, Hartwell PW (1986) The efficacy of sympathetic blockade in terminating acute herpes zoster and preventing the development of post-herpetic neuralgia. In: Rosberg B (ed) Proceedings from ESRA, Malmö, 1986.

Myofascial pain syndromes

For the most part the majority of myofascial pain syndromes are shortlived. They are caused by unusual muscular exertion or trauma and respond to the conservative therapy of rest and heat. However, there is a group of myofascial syndromes which are related to trigger points. These points are hyperirritable areas which can be associated with palpable bands of muscle tissue. Stimulation of this band of muscle tissue causes a burst of motor unit action potentials in the vicinity. This in turn is associated with pain at the site of stimulation as well as discrete and predictable areas of referred pain. These areas of muscle have previously been called fibrositis or fibrocytic nodules, muscular or nonarticular rheumatism, muscle hardening, etc. The areas of referred pain are predictable and have been mapped out in great detail. Of the multiple treatments designed for this disorder, local anesthetic and/or steroid injections into the nodule(s) appears to be the most effective. Similar results have, however, been obtained with injections of normal saline.

There are two basic methods of identifying the nodule/trigger zone:

1. Gentle manual palpation. A wide area is gently palpated with the left hand. It is often of great help if the palpating fingers and the area to be palpated are soaked with soap and water so that the palpating fingers can easily slide over the trigger zone area without exerting any major pressure. Firm pressure on the nodule typically causes the patient to complain bitterly about the pain.

2. Insertion of a needle into the suspect area. A positive identification would accentuate the patient's pain as well as its distal manifestations.

Injection of 1 – 2 ml of a solution containing 10 – 20 ml 0.25% bupivacaine and, for reinjections, 20 – 40 mg methylprednis-olone into the nodule through a 25 gauge needle is typically very painful. Usually several nodules are present, each of which should be injected. Sometimes a single set of injections will produce surprisingly long-lasting results. More often repeated injections are necessary. At follow-up, 70% – 80% of patients show good to excellent results. In most cases treatment should include physiotherapy.

Suggested reading

Brown BR Jr (1983) Myofascial and musculoskeletal pain. Int Anesthesiol Clin 21:139.

Frost FA, Toft B, Aaboe T (1984) Isotonic saline and methyl prednisolone acetate in blockade treatment of myofascial pain. Ugeskr Laeger 146:652

Kellgren JH (1938) Observation on referred pain arising from muscle. Clin Sci 3:175

Kellgren JH (1939) On the distribution of pain arising from deep somatic structures with charts of segmental pain areas. Clin Sci 4:35

Travell J, Rinzler SH (1952) The myofascial genesis of pain. Postgrad Med 11:425

Travell JG, Simons DG (1983) Myofascial pain and dysfunction: the trigger point manual. Williams & Wilkins, Baltimore.

Vascular disorders

Any vascular disease which causes decreased blood flow and ischemia can produce pain. At an advanced stage of the disease pain is present at rest while at a more moderate stage pain is related to exercise (intermittent claudication). Arteriosclerosis, diabetes, smoking Bürger's disease), embolism, and thrombosis are among the more common causes.

To this list must be added all of the pathologic phenomena that cause Raynaud's phenomenon. These include the causalgias and reflex sympathetic dystrophies. The pathologic feature common to all is a decreased peripheral blood flow with resulting pain. The mechanisms for this pain are quite complex and include a host of noxious substances liberated in the presence of hypoxemia.

The role of sympathetic block is twofold: (a) to ascertain whether destruction of the sympathetic nervous system, either with neurolytic solutions or by surgery, will increase blood flow and/or decrease symptomatology and (b) as an adjunct to surgical and medical procedures to promote peripheral blood flow.

In essence there are two types of clinical presentation that might occur:

1. The patient complaining of pain in whom decreased peripheral blood flow can easily be determined clinically or with laboratory tests

2. The patient who presents with pain only.

In the latter case an approach that could be used for a patient with bilateral lower extremity pain would be the following. After placement of an indwelling epidural catheter note the subjective effects of placebo and dilute local anesthetic drugs (0.25% lidocaine) which will give primarily a sympathetic nerve block. If the response of the patient is consistent and pain is relieved with the pharmacologically active agent and minimal to no relief is achieved with the placebo agent, it must then be determined whether sympathectomy should be the definitive treatment. This is accomplished by lumbar sympathetic blocks using active and inactive agents. If the patient's response is again appropriate then chemical or surgical sympathectomy is indicated.

An alternative to this is clinical evaluation based on the results obtained during a 5- to 7-day test period during which the patient is subjected to a continuous lumbar sympathetic block via an indwelling catheter. Alleviation of rest pain, improved walking distance, improved healing of ischemic ulcers, and delineation of gangrenous areas are all indications for a neurolytic sympathetic block.

In the first case, the situation is simpler. The effects of sympathetic block can be quantified using a variety of techniques including: (a) plethysmography, (b) clearance of radioactive substances, (c) temperature measurements, (d) Doppler flowmetry, (e) peripheral pH measurements, and (f) liquid crystal thermography. If the increase in blood flow is accompanied by improvement in pain and function, permanent sympathectomy is indicated.

The technique for lumbar sympathetic block has been described on p 142. Modifications when neurolytic agents are used would be the definite need for radiographic confirmation of needle placement. In addition, it is very useful to inject a small test dose of contrast medium, usually $0.1 - 0.25$ ml, which, if in the space between the psoas muscle and the body of the vertebra, will show a characteristic linear spread up and down this gutter. This should be followed by the injection of 6% – 10% phenol in contrast media, watching the spread of the solution as it is injected. At least three vertebral levels should be covered, which usually requires 2 – 5 ml of phenol mixture. A single needle technique is all that is required although some recommend the placement of two and occasionally three needles at the L2 – L4 level. A deliberate slow injection of phenol should be done in order to concentrate it around the nerves to be blocked. Also slow injection avoids spillage onto the somatic nerves, reducing the possibility of neuralgia.

Results

It should be emphasized that neurolytic sympathectomy is indicated only for arteriosclerotic disease in the foot of a leg not amenable to vascular surgery.

Rest pain is reported to be relieved in approximately 60% – 80%, gangrene improved in 40% – 50%, skin lesions in 35% – 60%, and claudication in 0% – 40%. Results are generally poorer in patients with diabetes and other small vessel diseases.

Complications

Neuralgia of the first lumbar nerve is reported to occur in up to 40%. This figure can be reduced if phenol is used instead of alcohol. The injection of a mixture of phenol and a radio-opaque medium under fluoroscopy is associated with an even lower risk of this complication. Duration of severe neuralgia is usually less than 2 months except following alcohol, where it may persist for longer.

Sensory loss, most commonly within the L1 distribution, is reported in approximately 5% of patients and may persist for up to 6 months but is rarely of any major importance.

Arterial hypotension and sexual dysfunction are extremely rare complications of lumbar neurolytic sympathectomy.

Fig. 4.3a. Lumbar sympathetic block, lateral view. The needle tip is placed at the anteriolateral aspect of the L_3 vertebral body and the injected contrast is seen to spread from L_2 to L_4.

Fig. 4.3b.

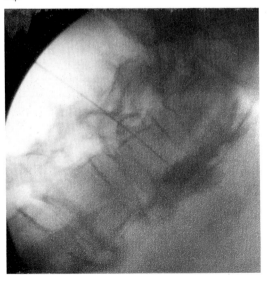

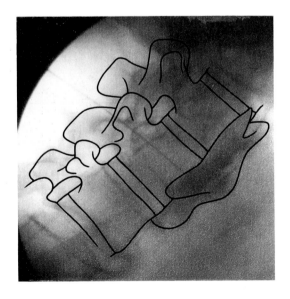

Suggested reading

Boas RA (1983) The sympathetic nervous system and pain relief. In: Swerdlow M (ed) Relief of intractable pain. Elsevier Scientific, Amsterdam, p 215

Cousins MJ, Reeve TS, Glynn CJ et al. (1979) Neurolytic lumbar sympathetic blockade: duration of denervation and relief of rest pain. Anaesth Intensive Care 7:121

Fyfe T, Quin RO (1975) Phenol sympathectomy in the treatment of intermittent claudication: a controlled clinical trial. Br J Surg 62:68

Hughes-Davies DI, Redman LR (1976) Chemical lumbar sympathectomy. Anaesthesia 31:1068

Löfström B, Zetterquist S (1969) Lumbar sympathetic blocks in the treatment of patients with obliterative arterial disease of the lower limb. Int Anesthesiol Clin 7:423

Pratt GH (1953) Anticoagulants and sympathetic nerve blocks in the treatment of vascular lesions. Effective therapeutic combination. JAMA 152:903

Reid W, Watt JK, Gray TG (1970) Phenol injection of the sympathetic chain. Br J Surg 57:45

Rose SS, Swerdlow M (1980) Pain due to peripheral vascular disease. In: Lipton S, (ed) Persistent pain: modern methods of treatment, vol 2. Academic Press, London, p 283

Skeehan TM, Cory PC Jr (1986) Neurolytic lumbar sympathetic block in the treatment of Raynaud's phenomenon. Anesthesiology 64:119

Volkmann J (1953) Über Zwischenfälle bei fast 70.000 Grenzstrangblockaden. Arch Klin Chir 273:750

Walsh JA, Glynn CJ, Cousins MJ et al (1984) Blood flow, sympathetic activity and pain relief following lumbar sympathetic blockade or surgical sympathectomy. Anaesth Intens Care 13:18

Phantom limb pain

Stump pain might develop postoperatively over several days to weeks. The skin over the stump grows excessively sensitive to touch. Burning sensations and muscle cramps are other symptoms which also are thought to be caused by physical irritation of cut nerves or neuromas.

The occurrence of phantom sensations after amputation is almost universal. For the most part the extent of the phantom diminishes with time and although many patients will state that they feel as though a part of the amputated extremity still remains, it exists in a nonpainful form. In fact with time the peripheral phantom often tends to recede into the stump itself. However, in 5% – 10% of cases the phantom is uncomfortable, the sensations variously being described as burning, shooting, cramp or crushing. These symptoms are more common in patients who prior to the amputation suffered pain in the limb. The symptoms usually remain for years and their intensity is strongly affected by variations of somatic input. Symptoms are often elicited from trigger zones which have a tendency to spread to healthy areas on the same or the opposite side.

Prior to treatment a differentiation must be made by the therapist between pain in the amputated extremity secondary to local causes in the stump such as neuroma or nerve entrapments, and more centrally located lesions. The approach to the patient with phantom limb pain must include a thorough examination of the stump and identification of hyperpathic points there. If these points can be identified then direct injection of a local anesthetic, with or without corticosteroids, small amounts of a neurolytic agent such as 5% – 7% phenol in water, or surgical resection may occasionally improve the situation. In many cases, however, these trigger zones cannot be identified.

The next step would be to do a spinal anesthetic to the T8–T10 level. If the phantom pain is relieved, differential blockade of lumbar somatic and sympathetic nerves might prove fruitful in delineating specific structures which could be ablated. Although this approach is theoretically sound, in reality very few patients can be relieved by neurodestructive procedures. Often the spinal is ineffective and one is left with supportive therapy only. Psychological methods have been reported to provide good results.

Suggested reading

Jensen TS, Krebs B, Nielsen J et al. (1985) Immediate and long-term phantom limb pain in amputees: incidence, clinical characteristics and relationship to pre-amputation limb pain. Pain 21:267

Melzack R (1971) Phantom limb pain: implications for treatment of pathologic pain. Anesthesiology 35:409

Sherman RA, Gall N, Gormly J (1979) Treatment of phantom limb pain with muscular relaxation training to disrupt the pain – anxiety – tension cycle. Pain 6:47

Chronic low back and ischialgic pain

Chronic low back pain and ischialgic pain are extremely common pain syndromes with a variety of etiologies, of which many are poorly understood or unknown. Therapy includes medication, surgery, physical therapy, manipulation, traction, hyperstimulation analgesia, nerve blocks, chemonucleolysis, and steroid injections.

Suggested reading

Flor H, Turk DC (1984) Ethiological theories and treatments for chronic back pain. I. Somatic models and interventions. Pain 19:105

Lewinnek GE (1978) Management of low back pain and sciatica. Int Anesthesiol Clin 21:61

Sedzimir CB (1980) Lumbo-sacral root pain. In: Lipton S (ed) Persistent pain: modern methods of treatment, vol 2. Academic Press, London, p 143

Turk DC, Flor H (1984) Etiological theories and treatments for chronic back pain. II. Psychological models and interventions. Pain 19:209

Epidural/spinal injections

Epidural/spinal injections are only symptomatic treatment and should only be performed after adequate workup to exclude infection or a space-occupying lesion as the cause of the patient's symptoms. Injections should be supplemented by physiotherapy and physical training aimed at improving the strength of the abdominal and paravertebral muscles and general physical activity.

The use of epidural/spinal injections of normal saline or dilute local anesthetics alone or in combination with corticosteroids, employing intermittent or continuous techniques in this context, is still very controversial. Several studies have shown rather similar results indicating beneficial effects of this therapy. Only a limited number have been controlled, however, and most of these show nonsignificant differences between control and experimental groups.

A variety of minor transient complications are reported. Major complications include epidural abscess, meningitis, arachnoiditis, and permanent paralysis.

Considering the very doubtful curative effects and the incidence of complications we recommend a conservative approach.

In patients who have had pain for more than 3 months despite adequate medical treatment and have not previously undergone laminectomy ("virgin backs"), a segmental epidural employing corticosteroids only or, for patients in severe pain, mixed with minimal amounts of a local anesthetic (3 – 5 ml of 0.5% bupivacaine), may be tried. In previously operated patients the situation is much more complex and epidural/spinal injections are far less successful than in "virgin backs." We recommend that this therapy be used cautiously in such patients.

Suggested reading

Benzon HT (1986) Epidural steroid injections for low back pain and lumbosacral radiculopathy. Pain 24:277

Cuckler JM, Bernini PA, Wiesel SW et al. (1985) The use of epidural steroids in the treatment of lumbar radicular pain. J Bone Joint Surg 67A:63

Kepes ER, Duncalf D (1985) Treatment of backache with spinal injections of local anesthetics, spinal and systemic steroids. A review. Pain 22:33

Miller RD, Munger WL, Powell PE (1980) Chronic pain and local anesthetic neural blockade. In: Cousins MJ, Bridenbaugh PO, (eds) Neural blockade in clinical anesthesia and management of pain. JB Lippincott, Philadelphia, p 628

Steinberger EK, Urban BJ, France RD (1984) Partial blindness and chest pain following epidural steroid blocks. Reg Anesth 9:98

Local injections

The multiple etiologies of chronic low back pain include myofascial pain. In many cases considerable relief can be obtained after injection of trigger zones as described on p 182. The trigger zones can be difficult to localize so the utmost patience is recommended during careful examination of the muscles of the patient's back. Injections of small volumes of local anesthetics, plain or mixed with corticosteroids or even an antifibrinolytic (10 mg triamcinolone), have been recommended.

Suggested reading

Bourne IHL (1979) Treatment of backache with local injection. Practitioner 222:708

Sonne M, Christensen K, Hansen SE et al (1985) Injection of steriods and local anaesthetics as therapy for low-back pain. J Rheumatol 14:343

Facet joint injections

Facet abnormalities can account for many of the symptoms in low back pain even when associated with leg pain and paresthesias. Classical symptoms of the facet syndrome are unilateral hip and buttock pain, cramping pain in the leg above the knee, and low back stiffness. The typical signs are local paralumbar tenderness, pain on spine hyperextension, absence of neurologic deficit or signs of root tension, and elicitation of pain in hip, buttock, or back by straight leg raising.

The facet and its capsule are innervated by the three branches of the medial branch of the posterior primary ramus of the spinal nerve. Each medial branch supplies at least three facet joints. It is rarely possible to perform diagnostic or therapeutic nerve blocks of the medial branch. Facet joint injections, on the other hand, provide up to 40% good to excellent results.

The patient is placed in a 30 – 45° prone position. A 7.5- to 10-cm 22 gauge needle is inserted 2 – 3 cm from the midline between the appropriate spinous processes under infiltration of a dilute local anesthetic. It is passed in a perpendicular manner toward the joint until it hits bone. It is then "walked" in a fanwise manner into the joint, which one notices by a rubbery give. The procedure should be performed under fluoroscopic control which also verifies the correct positioning of the needle tip intra-articularly. Each joint is injected with 2 ml of a solution made up of 9 ml 0.25% bupivacaine and 1 ml (40 mg) methylprednisolone. Conventionally the three lowermost facet joints are injected unilaterally if pain is unilateral, but otherwise bilaterally. The procedure is safe provided subarachnoid or intravascular needle position is ruled out, and can be performed on an outpatient basis.

Suggested reading

Lippitt AB (1984) The facet joint and its role in spine pain. Management with facet joint injections. Spine 9:746

Lynch MC, Tayler JF (1986) Facet joint injection for low back pain. A clinical study. J Bone Joint Surg (Br) 68:138

Post-traumatic pain syndromes

Trauma is ordinarily followed by healing of the wound, cessation of pain, return of function, etc. Occasionally healing does not take place in this predictable manner, and increasing pain and loss of function occur.

Causalgia

This often extremely painful syndrome was given its name by Mitchell in 1867. According to the International Association for the Study of Pain it is defined as a syndrome of sustained burning pain after a traumatic nerve lesion combined with vasomotor and sudomotor dysfunction and later trophic changes. The pain and dysesthesia are not restricted to the area supplied by the injured nerve but are mostly present in the peripheral portions of the extremity. The symptoms appear and may reach a maximum soon after the injury and may persist for decades if not properly treated. The dysesthesias may be so intense that the patient cannot wear his clothes, physiotherapy cannot be performed, the patient protects his painful limb constantly, and, in some cases, suicide is contemplated.

Causalgia minor

This syndrome has a less dramatic symptomatology and is frequently not caused by direct neural trauma. It may occur secondary to fractures, crush injury, operative trauma, and even minor trauma such as cuts, sprains, or falls. In some cases it is secondary to the shoulder – hand syndrome and in other cases secondary to unknown causes. Due to the multiple origins it has appeared in the literature under a variety of names such as post-traumatic sympathetic dystrophy, reflex sympathetic dystrophy, Sudeck's dystrophy, post-traumatic dystrophy, and sympathetic neurovascular dystrophy. The diagnosis should be suspected when at least three of the following six symptoms are observed in the limb:

1. Persistent generalized burning pain
2. Edema
3. Radiographic evidence of demineralization
4. Cyanosis
5. Hyperhidrosis
6. Hyperesthesia to light touch

The diagnosis is confirmed by various measurements of the cutaneous temperature, regional blood flow, or psychogalvanic reflex response.

For over 50 years sympathetic blocks have been the most reliable diagnostic test and sympathectomy, chemical or surgical, the most reliable therapeutic measure.

In case of relief of symptoms, often of an interval well beyond the duration of the block itself, repetitive blocks should be performed until the pain is controlled. The technique of stellate ganglion block (for the upper extremity) has been described on p 128, and that of lumbar sympathetic block (for the lower extremity) on p 142.

If relief from repeated sympathetic blocks becomes less effective or static and the initial response is dramatic but of short duration, surgical sympathectomy (for the upper extremity) or neurolysis of the lumbar sympathetic ganglia for the lower extremity) should be considered. It is our experience that repeated blocks with local anesthetics suffice in most cases, although in rare cases, they have to be repeated 20 or more times.

It is of utmost importance that the nerve block therapy is combined with adequate and intense physiotherapy, preferably within the pain clinic area. If repeated sympathetic blocks are begun within 6 months after first appearance of symptoms, more than 80% of patients will be relieved of their symptoms while the functional recovery is reported to be less good. Results in cases with a duration of 6 – 12 months or longer have been reported as relatively poor, although other reports claim favorable results even in cases of long standing.

Suggested reading

Boas RA (1983) The sympathetic nervous system and pain relief. In: Swerdlow M (ed) Relief of intractable pain. Elsevier Scientific, Amsterdam, p 219

Bonica JJ (1979) Causalgia and other reflex sympathetic dystrophies. In: Bonica JJ, Liebeskind JC, Albe-Fessard DE, (eds) Advances in pain research and therapy, vol 3. Raven Press, New York, p 141

Carron H, Weller R. (1974) Post-traumatic sympathetic dystrophy. Adv Neurol 4:485

Martelete M (1983) Comparative results in the treatment of causalgia and other reflex sympathetic dystrophies. In: Yokota T, Dubner R, (eds) Current topics in pain research and therapy. Proceedings of the international symposium on pain. Kyoto, December 12–13, 1982. Excerpta Medica, Amsterdam, p 249

Mitchell SW, Morehouse GR, Keen WW (1864) Gunshot wounds and other injuries of nerves. JB Lippincott, Philadelphia, p 164

Nathan PW (1983) Pain and the sympathetic nervous system. In: Yokota T, Dubner R, (eds) Current topics in pain research and therapy. Proceedings of the international symposium on pain. Kyoto, December 12–13, 1982. Excerpta Medica, Amsterdam, p 241

Patman RD, Thompson JE, Persson AV (1973) Management of post-traumatic pain syndromes: report of 113 cases. Ann Surg 177:780

Procacci P, Francini F, Zoppi M et al. (1975) Cutaneous pain threshold changes after sympathetic block in reflex dystrophies. Pain 1:167

Ramamurthy S, Winnie AP (1985) Regional anesthetic techniques for pain relief. Semin Anesth 4:237

Roberts WJ (1986) A hypothesis on the physiological basis for causalgia and related pains. Pain 24:297

Sunderland S (1976) Pain mechanisms in causalgia. J Neurol Neurosurg Psychiatry 39:471

Wall PD, Gutnick M (1974) Ongoing activity in peripheral nerves: the physiology and pharmacology of impulses originating from a neuroma. Exp Neurol 43:580

Wang JK, Erickson RP, Ilstrup DM (1985) Repeated stellate ganglion blocks for upper-extremity reflex sympathetic dystrophy. Reg Anesth 10:125

5. Debatable applications

Introduction

The authors reviewed both the older and more recent literature and concluded that the following unusual indications for nerve block therapy were worthy of presentation in this book. One could argue that additional disorders should be included here or even perhaps that those chosen were inappropriate.

We do not wish to suggest that regional techniques should be the prime therapy employed for the conditions discussed below but rather include this section because we think it is of interest. In addition the listed conditions are frequently present in patients about to undergo surgery. The concomitant disease might be an indication for a regional block – alone or in combination with light general anesthesia – in the anesthesiologic management of the patient.

Asthma and status asthmaticus

The basic treatment for asthma and status asthmaticus is medical. However, throughout the last half century, anecdotal reports and series of cases have appeared in the medical literature noting the effects of various types of nerve block technique in providing symptomatic relief in patients with acute asthma and status asthmaticus.

A variety of surgical attacks on the autonomic nervous system have been tried in order to reduce the frequency and severity of asthmatic attacks, with variable success. These procedures have included glomectomy (removal of the carotid body), stellate ganglionectomy, thoracic ganglionectomy, and surgical lysis of both sympathetic and vagal fibers, but they are no longer performed.

The innervation of the lung contains both parasympathetic and sympathetic efferent and afferent fibers. The parasympathetic vagal efferent fibers are felt to be primarily bronchoconstrictor whereas the sympathetic fibers are primarily bronchodilator. It would seem that block of the parasympathetic fibers would be effective for treating bronchospasm. However, clinical experience seems to indicate that block of the sympathetic fibers is useful in a certain number of cases. Block procedures which have been used successfully include stellate ganglion block, thoracic paravertebral block, and thoracic epidural block.

When used in the acute situation or when the patient is in status asthmaticus all authors present a certain success rate in which the acute condition was completely reversed with restoration of normal breathing patterns, relaxation of chest wall spasm, and a rapid liquefaction and elimination of secretions. In fact, in the Bromage book on epidural anesthesia a thoracic epidural block from T2 to T10 apparently proved life-saving in a patient who was approaching death during an acute asthmatic episode despite all therapy, including deep ether anesthesia. Within a short period after epidural block the patient, who was comatose, awoke, PCO^2 fell from the 90–100 torr level to 60 torr, and the patient could be extubated and was talking and alert within 2 h.

This type of a report, plus many others in the literature, suggests that block therapy might be of some use when medical treatment is an obvious failure. Due to the addition of very potent bronchodilators and other remedies this is now rarely the case.

Thoracic epidural analgesia might, however, be used for intraoperative as well as postoperative analgesia in patients with bronchial asthma.

Coronary insufficiency – angina pectoris

Anginal pain is most often treated pharmacologically by agents that reduce cardiac work and/or myocardial oxygen demand or improve myocardial oxygen supply. Recent pharmacologic advances have contributed considerably to a successful outcome of medical therapy. Another important step forward in therapy was the introduction of coronary artery bypass procedures.

In the past sympathetic blockade or surgical or neurolytic sympathectomy was used in the treatment of patients with severe angina pectoris. Even today, we cannot let statements such as "one of the outstanding and most brilliant chapters in the history of analgesic block therapy for the management of pain has been the use of paravertebral alcohol injections for definitive treatment of angina pectoris" (quoted from Bonica) go unnoticed. There are still occasional patients who suffer considerable pain and/or anxiety from angina pectoris in spite of optimal attempts at medical and surgical therapy. This can be illustrated by the following case:

A 46-year old man suffered myocardial infarctions in 1980 and 1981. In 1982 he underwent a triple aortocoronary bypass procedure which initially relieved him from frequent retrosternal pain. However, severe angina pectoris reappeared 1 month later and subsequent coronary angiograms revealed occlusion of the grafts. Immediate reoperation was rejected due to poor left ventricular function and enlargement of the heart. He suffered almost constant retrosternal pain, even at rest, aggravated by very mild physical strain such as brushing his teeth and dressing. Because of the frequent attacks of pain which continued despite comprehensive medical therapy, he made multiple visits to the emergency room, where even standard doses of morphine did not help. At this stage he was referred to the pain clinic and an epidural catheter was inserted at the T3–4 interspace. Injection of 3 ml of 0.5% bupivacaine was followed by pain relief and mild exercise did not elicit angina pectoris. Systolic arterial blood pressure fell by 10–15 torr. Radionucleotide investigations of left ventricular function did not show any changes as compared with conditions prior to the block. After comprehensive instructions to the patient and his wife he was sent home for self-administration of epidural injections of 2 ml (later 4 ml) of 0.5% bupivacaine, which relieved anginal pain for about 4 months. Originally he would require four to six injections per day. Signs of tachyphylaxis appeared during the fourth month. Epidural morphine, 1–2 mg every 8–12 h was substituted and proved equally effective for a time. Bilateral neurolysis of the T1 – T5 sympathetic ganglia was then performed under radiologic control in two stages employing 2 ml of absolute alcohol per ganglion, with good pain relief for 3–5 months.

For emergency treatment of severe anginal pain when medical therapies have failed a left stellate ganglion block might be performed. It should be remembered that the afferents from the heart pass through the cardiac nerves, going to the lower and middle cervical ganglion primarily on the left side.

Myocardial infarction

There are a number of anecdotal reports of beneficial effects of high thoracic epidural anesthesia in patients with acute myocardial infarction but only one of a more comprehensive nature, published in Russian. The material consisted of 300 patients with "large focus" myocardial infarction, of whom 110 showed signs of cardiac failure on admission and 96 various arrhythmias. High thoracic epidural anesthesia was induced shortly after admission. All patients experienced complete pain relief within 5 – 10 min. Their systolic arterial blood pressure was reduced by 10 – 15 torr and the heart rate by six to eight beats per minute. Pulmonary edema subsided in five of 10 patients. Electrocardiographic ST elevations were normalized in 30 patients. Respiratory acidosis and/or arterial hypoxemia returned to acceptable levels in all patients. Arrhythmias disappeared in 27 of 96 patients. No episode of ventricular arrhythmia was observed in any patient, while sinus bradycardia occurred in ten and significant arterial hypotension in eight patients. The author concluded that high thoracic epidural anesthesia in acute myocardial infarction has an antiarrhythmic effect and provides complete freedom from pain. The presence of arterial hypotension and/or AV block should be considered relative contraindications to this technique.

Suggested reading

Bonica JJ (1953) The management of pain. Lea and Febiger, Philadelphia, p 1327

Tevelenok YA (1977) Peridural anaesthesia in the acute period of myocardial infarction (in Russian). Anesteziologija I Reanimatologija 3:36

Pulmonary edema

Effective ways of treating the pulmonary edema secondary to heart failure by means of chemical sympathectomy via a thoracic or lumbar epidural block have been known for 40 years but for the most part have been lost in the shuffle as new medical treatments have proved very efficacious. However, in cases of intractable pulmonary edema this form of therapy should be considered. Mechanisms involved may be more than shifts of circulating blood volume out of the lungs into a dilated peripheral vascular system. It has been shown that there is also some direct arterial vasodilatation in the lungs after the blocks.

Cardiospasm

Spasm is a fairly common disorder of the lower esophagus and in a high percentage of cases causes some substernal distress which may radiate to the back or neck. A functional disorder of muscles of the distal esophagus appears to occur in association with psychological problems.

In intractable cases, paravertebral sympathetic blocks from T5 to T8 bilaterally or a segmental epidural may provide symptomatic relief by causing relaxation of the circular muscle fibers of the cardiac sphincter. Often relief lasts far longer than the actual duration of the block.

Suggested reading

De Sousa Pereira A (1946) Blocking of the splanchnic nerves and the first lumbar sympathetic ganglion. Technic, accidents and clinical indications. Arch Surg 53:32

Index